DR. WILLIAMS-NGIRWA'S
THE POWER OF A SMILE

DR. WILLIAMS-NGIRWA'S
THE POWER OF A SMILE

How Complete Health Dentistry is *Revolutionizing America*

DONNA R. WILLIAMS-NGIRWA, DDS

WITH: Charles Whitney, M.D.
Michael L. Gelb, DDS, MS
Gina L. Pritchard, MSN, RN, CNS, ACNP, DNPc

THE COMPLETE HEALTH PRACTICE SERIES

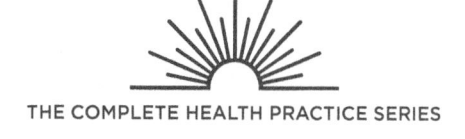

Copyright © 2018 by NextLevel Practice.

All rights reserved. No part of this book may be used or reproduced in any manner whatsoever without prior written consent of the author, except as provided by the United States of America copyright law.

Printed in the United States of America.

This publication is designed to provide accurate and authoritative information in regard to the subject matter covered. It is sold with the understanding that the publisher is not engaged in rendering legal, accounting, or other professional services. If legal advice or other expert assistance is required, the services of a competent professional person should be sought.

TABLE OF CONTENTS

Chapter 1 1
THE POWER OF A SMILE

Chapter 2 15
A REVOLUTION TAKES ROOT

Chapter 3 27
INFLAMMATION: THE SILENT KILLER

Chapter 4 37
THE HEART OF THE MATTER

Chapter 5 49
DON'T FORGET

Chapter 6 59
AN INFLAMED BODY IS A SICK BODY

Chapter 7 69
THE POWER OF A GOOD NIGHT'S SLEEP

Chapter 8 79
BABIES, BELLIES, AND BLOOD SUGAR

Chapter 9 89
THE COST OF DOING NOTHING IS TOO GREAT

Chapter 10 95
THE COMPLETE HEALTH DENTISTRY® TRANSFORMATION

CHAPTER 1

THE POWER OF A SMILE

"Rule number one: save the tooth at all costs."
That's what my professor told a lecture hall full of first-year dental students back in 1986. She said that you should never pull a tooth until you've explored every possible alternative. We were taught about the difficulties people suffered with while having to use false teeth and that fillings, root canals, crowns, and bridges were designed to restore function to a patient whose overall health would be diminished if we removed teeth without replacing them. We were taught that those dental prostheses could in no way replace a natural tooth.

After I heard that, I cracked open a new notebook, grabbed a freshly-sharpened pencil, and jotted down this first principle of dentistry. Then I looked up to see beautiful images of a perfect smile projected onto the lecture hall wall.

It was in school where we learned about how important teeth and a beautiful smile is in making a great first impression—how teeth were absolutely essential and an integral part of the digestive process. We learned how important the teeth are for speaking and forming words properly—even how important they are for protection.

In Tanzania, you can experience the breathtakingly beautiful peaks of Mount Kilimanjaro, the third highest mountain in the world, then step onto the brilliant white sands and the bluest waters of Zanzibar. There's the ferocious, natural beauty of Tanzania's Serengeti, the Ngorongoro Crater, Lake Manyara, and other national parks—but it becomes quite a dichotomy to then travel three days on a dusty train ride to get up country to rural Tanzania. We passed hundreds of people, some getting on and off the train, some just selling their wares as we went by. Children often pretended to chase the train until they couldn't keep up any longer.

We would travel far into the rural villages and see the despair of rural people who have limited access to the basic necessities that we in the United States take for granted.

It was in the summer of 1987 when I found myself in a rural African village, extracting teeth for the very first time. The Shinyanga Region in Tanzania had a ratio of eight hundred thousand people to one dentist. When we went to the dental clinic in the morning, there were people lined up, waiting to relieve their pain. It was toward the end of that first day that I counted the number of extractions—fifty teeth.

My first day operating on actual patients, I extracted fifty teeth. I certainly honed my extraction skills in the Regional Hospital in Shinyanga Tanzania. But, I was faced with another dichotomy—extracting teeth that I knew were savable versus getting people out of their immediate tooth pain. The next day, I extracted fifty-one teeth. I made a mental note to myself; I had an abundance of gratitude of having the experience working alongside Dr. Kishai and learning how to perform extractions with ease, but I felt a distinct sadness that these individuals would be left with fewer teeth to chew. I felt like I was creating a lifetime of subsequent dental problems, though at that moment, they had no other options—no other way to relieve one of the most excruciating of pains: dental pain.

Within an hour of sunrise, we had more patients lined up than an American dentist sees in a week. And more were on their way—some with gum disease, some with cavities, and infections; all of them in extraordinary pain. But there wasn't time for fillings. There wasn't time for root canals. And there sure as heck wasn't time for cleanings. We needed to treat excruciating pain, stop the spread of infections, and move on as quickly as we could. No time for oral health education. Which meant that all we could do was pull teeth.

Pull teeth. Pull teeth. Pull teeth.

We were doing the best we could with the resources we had, but we certainly weren't doing a good job. In fact, we were doing a decidedly bad job. We may have been treating infections, but we were also turning our patients into dental cripples by pulling their teeth.

After two days with that mission, I swore to myself that I would find a better way. And not just a better way to serve Tanzanian patients, but a better way to serve patients around the world. Because dentists neglect their patients everywhere, America included.

Sure, not all dentists perform fifty extractions a day. But the vast majority of American dentists don't look at the big picture. They treat the individual symptoms in front of them—cavities, cracked teeth, swollen gums—and they miss the underlying causes. They become tooth mechanics and gum gardeners. They don't treat whole bodies, they don't treat whole people, and they do virtually nothing to prevent disease.

But it doesn't have to be that way. In dental school, you learn about anatomy, physiology, microbiology, biochemistry, pharmacology—we learn everything about the mouth being part of the whole body. It is in the last two years of dental school that we focus solely on the mouth and oftentimes forget that there is an entire body connected to that mouth. Back when I was in dental school, I believed that we could do better. Now I know it for a fact.

My obsession with oral health care began in high school, the day I got braces. I was lying in the patient chair, waiting for the orthodontist, when I looked over to my right and saw a tray full of equipment and instruments. Different cements and medicaments— such an array of different items that I became very curious. For some teenagers, that image probably would have inspired extraordinary dread. But for me, all it inspired was excitement. I had always loved working with my hands— cooking, playing piano, anything that is creative. So, to me, those instruments just looked like fun. I was intrigued by the doctors who got to use them—got to clean and craft with them, and make beautiful smiles. I have always had a leaning toward going into the health care field and being able to creatively use your hands was so interesting to me.

I decided to spend part of my senior year of high school interning for a local dentist. That internship would mark my first encounter in a major way working in a dental office. I loved how a dentist could take a person with broken down and missing teeth and create a beautiful smile. However, it seemed the job was monotonous— all the dentist did was clean teeth and gums and fill cavities. Clean gums. Fill cavities. Clean gums. Fill cavities. All day. Every day. All year. Every year.

Like most interns, I was often asked to work at the reception desk. And instead of feeling misused or underutilized, I actually felt grateful for the opportunity. His patients fascinated me. From the reception desk, I could reel them into conversations about their day to day lives.

After the internship concluded, my next internship was at WINX Radio Station in Maryland. I just figured that I wanted to work in a field that involved meeting people, learning about their lives, telling stories, and travel. I wanted to work in a field that encouraged developing relationships. I wanted to travel the world and meet different people and understand their lives. So, I started out my undergraduate education in the School of Communications at Howard University in Washington, DC.

Since then, I've learned that those desires and instincts make me a better dentist. I've learned that the best dentists don't hole themselves up in their offices. In fact, the world has been opened up to me as a result of dentistry. They get in cars, on trains, boats, and on planes, and they bring oral health care to communities that don't have it yet. I've learned that the best dentists don't just treat canines and molars. They treat whole bodies and whole people. And I've learned that the best dentists do more than drilling and filling. They're always on the lookout for new ways that dentistry can help their patients.

Still, I'm grateful for both internships because it made me the doctor I am today. Because of that experience, I decided not to pursue dentistry after high school. Instead, I spent the first part of college studying communications. And when I did course-correct back toward oral health care, I studied dental hygiene first before going to dental school. Without those two landmark periods of learning, I wouldn't have had the skills to run the holistic practice that I run today, and I wouldn't have known how to advocate for a better, more complete approach to dentistry.

I graduated in 1990 from Baltimore College of Dental Surgery, University of Maryland, the first dental school in the world. My first practice was in Charlotte Amalie, Unites States Virgin Island. Afterward, I moved to New York and opened Morningside Dental

Care. The office began as a run of the mill dental office, serving patients in New York and the vicinity with comprehensive, but standard bread and butter dentistry. It wasn't until the birth of my son, Sadiki, that dentistry for me was turned on its head.

My son came into the world as a two pounds, one ounce, twenty-six-week-old premature infant, and it wasn't immediately clear how long he would stay. The problem was a simple one to explain, and a difficult one to fix: he couldn't breathe. He stayed in the hospital for four months in the Neonatal Intensive Care Unit (NICU) so his lungs would develop and he could breathe on his own.

Eventually, the doctors cleared Sadiki to go home. We were sent home with a pulse oximeter and a CPAP. I was a first-time mother which was intimidating enough, and then there was hospital equipment on top of that. And if that wasn't enough, the very night we brought him home, our baby boy was turning blue. He couldn't breathe. We sped back to the hospital, where he stayed an additional two weeks.

A few hours later, the doctors told us that our baby had picked up a Strep A infection while in the hospital before he left. Eventually, he got better and was sent home. But even then, every night for the next two and a half years, he slept with the CPAP and pulse oximeter. My nights for the first few years were harrowing. I would place the CPAP on him as he fell asleep. Then I would fall asleep. After a few hours in the night, he would inadvertently take it off, the pulse oximeter monitor would alarm, then I would wake up startled and put the CPAP mask back on. This was the routine that we had developed. During the first few years, there was little sleep for either of us, and we feared for his life—how was he going to survive and grow? Sadiki was hospitalized nine times over the course of the next two years, and was intubated six of those times.

It was what I learned during one of the hospitalizations that forever changed how I think of medicine, dentistry, and health in general. I have a number of family members who are physicians, and have always looked up to them and was inspired by them. I thought it was the physicians that cured patients. However, I soon learned better.

It was during one of those hospitalizations with Sadiki at Mount Sinai Hospital in New York City that he coded. The alarms rang, the nurses screamed, "Code blue, code blue!" The doctors all ran into the room and moved me out. I was frantic. They called a chaplain to my side to ensure that I had spiritual support. Just after it happened, I frantically pleaded to the resident who cared for him to help my son and make him better. It was during this moment that the resident informed me that, "as physicians, we can support the airway with our machines, but the body has to heal itself."

And now, twenty years later, little Sadiki is a beautifully, healthy 6'3" 190-pound communications major in college—go figure. I am so blessed. It's not too late for him to choose dentistry if he wants.

That resident gave me two gifts: the first gift—the greatest gift I've ever been given—was the gift of my son, alive and healthy. And the second gift was that kernel of wisdom, which flipped my understanding of medicine inside out: "The body needs to heal itself." You need to be able to breathe. Breathing is everything—breathing is life.

From that moment to this one, I've oriented my career around the philosophy that doctors don't heal people. Doctors help people heal themselves. From what we put into our body (diet), to our mental health and exercise are critical to creating that foundation. And the most important thing is we need is to breathe. Breathing is life, and most importantly, it all stems from the mouth!

As a dentist, it's my job to get to know the insides of my patients' mouths. Which makes me both the chief lookout and the first line of defense when it comes to diagnosing and treating conditions that block airways (in chapter seven, we'll look at those conditions in more detail). It also puts me in a privileged position to prevent, diagnose, and treat oral conditions that contribute to systemic illnesses such as diabetes, heart attacks, stroke, and dementia.

This philosophy has motivated me to take copious hours of continuing education classes so we can expand what our dental practice offers. It inspired me to study and receive a fellowship in natural dentistry as well as a preceptorship in the Bale/Doneen Method. It's inspired me to host a radio show about oral health care, to train my entire team in Complete Health Dentistry®. Our entire team must be able to educate our patients about how oral health is connected to overall health. It inspired me to petition governor Andrew Cuomo of the State of New York to recognize February as Gum Disease Awareness Month, and to invest in procedures and equipment that most dentists would rather not bother with.

Our CBCT cone beam takes three-dimensional x-rays of patients' heads and necks. Not only can we place implants more accurately and find additional canals in a tooth, but we can also evaluate the airway so we can see if the nasal passage, sinuses, tongue, or palate might impinge upon the space, making it more difficult to breathe. It also can catch calcifications in the arteries that cause blockages. We may use diet analysis to find out exactly what a patient is eating that may be contributing to their disease, and to help patients halt the progress of diabetes, gum disease, and tooth decay before it's too late. We've made the move to more bio-compatible materials, and have removed mercury fillings from the office about eighteen years ago. You see, mercury is toxic, and those traditional fillings could potentially be made of up to 50 percent mercury. Overtime, they also can cause teeth to fracture. Digital x-rays are just the standard we use all the time which reduces radiation exposure by about 80 percent.

Of course, none of this will matter if people don't go to the dentist. So we also invest in treatment strategies that make office visits faster and more comfortable. Instead of treating gum disease the old-fashioned way—cutting gums open, cleaning the teeth, and sewing gums back together again—I was trained by Millennium Dental in the LANAP Therapy (Laser Assisted New Attachment Procedure) and then invested in cutting-edge laser technology that reduces pain, expedites procedures, and dramatically improves the results. This is the only FDA approved method for true periodontal regeneration. We also use it to save failing implants. In fact, I was the second dentist in New York City to be trained in this specific procedure.

This work changes lives. One of our patients had been told that her gum disease was so bad, she was going to have to have all her teeth pulled out. Then she found us. And fifteen years later, she has healthier gums, a healthier body, and all of her original teeth. In fact, most of our patients who have had LANAP surgery share the same story, then after surgery they have significant improvements with stronger, healthier teeth, and improved overall health—they end up saving teeth that had previously been condemned.

And while I'm working hard to save teeth and prevent extractions here in the States, I'm also working to honor the commitment that I made decades ago in Tanzania.

Back in 1981, my parents founded a non-profit organization called AHEAD Inc. (Adventures in Health, Education, and Agricultural Development Inc.), which was devoted to improving health care and education in Tanzania and the Gambia. Today, I'm on their board of directors, and I make trips to Tanzania every year. In fact, my three siblings and their spouses are on the board of directors—some of them for more than thirty years. Throughout the years, AHEAD Inc. has made many achievements, particularly working in the rural areas hand in hand and in partnership with the villagers.

At AHEAD Inc., I see my future as working to launch an oral and disease prevention program that will focus on ending the practice of extractions and focus on placing sealants. It will also focus on oral health education, diet, and to prevent incidents of decay that become more rampant as people in developing countries have increased access to processed food which includes a lot of sugar. To solve the problem of x-ray scarcity, digital x-rays make it so that you never have x-ray shortages again, and in fact, it is much better for the patient.

AHEAD Inc.'s ultimate goal is to establish infrastructure in the communities we work in and to support people in the village. "Helping people help themselves" is part of our mission statement. We believe that education is the key to achieving that goal, so one of our most recent projects focused on renovating a school. First things first, we overhauled their women's bathroom, which had been falling part. (Things had gotten so bad that the women were using the bushes instead of the toilets.) And then we got to work wiring the school with electricity so students would be able to see the chalkboard when the day is overcast as well as being able to study after dark while still at school.

Another one of our projects began with the idea of building a pediatric ward and isolation unit. When the community rallied around the effort, they drew in government support and helped us elevate the mission. Now this little project to build a pediatric ward has become a huge initiative to build a health center with the community themselves taking the lead on the entire project—it is becoming a model project for others to emulate.

And I'm not the only person in my office doing this kind of work. I like to say that our Morningside Dental team is a little United Nations. Together, we represent a diverse array of countries and cultures. And each of us has become a Complete Health® ambassador to our respective communities. Together, we're working to spread our philosophy of preventative, holistic health care around the world, from the Caribbean to the Philippines, from Cuba to India to Russia, Colombia, and the United States of America, to name a few countries that we represent.

We are so fortunate to have our office in Harlem, in New York City. Harlem is so diverse and the neighborhood is truly a melting pot. People from so many different countries, cultures, races, and religions, all living together. It's just beautiful. Morningside Dental Care is a reflection of that, and the patients we are honored to care for reflect that wonderful diversity. So it happens quite frequently that patients suffering from gum disease and tooth decay reflect back on their lives in their home countries, remembering that before they moved to the United States, they had perfect oral health. They learn the hard way that when a person moves, it's not just their address that changes. Diets change too, and it's usually for the worse.

There's a high cost of convenience in America, where the most accessible foods are processed. They're full of unnatural, addictive fats and sugars—ingredients designed in laboratories, not grown on farms. So it's hardly a surprise when we see new citizens—particularly from Africa, the Caribbean, South and Central America—experience increased oral health challenges that they did not have prior to moving to this country.

In the African American community, preventable chronic illnesses have become commonplace: diabetes, obesity, strokes, heart diseases, Alzheimer's, and periodontal diseases. And we can't blame it all on genetic pre-dispositions. It's as much about the practices that we inherit as it is about the genes that we inherit.

We need to start making more trips to physicians and dentists and focus on prevention. We need to stop playing catch-up when it comes to health care. We can take the lead.

Yet these conditions aren't unique to the African American community. The reality is that they're universal. Which is why each and every one of us needs to practice preventative health care. We need to be proactive about caring for ourselves. Because preventing illnesses is much easier and much more affordable than treating illnesses.

That's why we need to stop framing preventative health care as a privilege of the elite. Your race, your income, your country of origin—none of these things should factor into how you think about your health. Preventative health care isn't more expensive—it saves you money in the long run. Yet, in our society that needs everything in an instant, it can be more challenging to practice. It requires commitment. But you and your family's lives are worth that extra effort.

Committing to taking a holistic approach to your health isn't just about protecting yourself either. It's about protecting the people you love by staying healthy for them—by showing up for them. And it's about passing a tradition of good health on to your children.

The mouth is the gateway to the body. If the mouth is diseased, the body will follow. By keeping your gums and your teeth healthy, you can keep your whole body healthy. In the chapters that follow, I'm going to demonstrate exactly that. You'll see for yourself how a holistic, complete approach to your oral health care can change—and even save—your life.

Tupac Shakur once wrote a poem "The Power of a Smile." He wrote about all the powers that conspire to hurt us: the power of guns, the power of fire, the power of anger. But at the end of that poem, he named the one power that can save us: "The power of a smile," he wrote, "can heal a frozen heart."

Your smile is so important, yet too often we take it for granted. The smile is where people make the first impression of you. It can help you land that ideal job or find your perfect mate. Chewing, digestion, speaking, protection—even the very act of breathing to keep us alive—takes place in the mouth. If you care for your smile, it can have a tremendous impact on the hearts of the people around you. And it can also have a tremendous impact on your own heart.

I'm sure that Tupac meant that figuratively. But I don't. I mean it literally. Read on, and you'll see why.

CHAPTER 2

A REVOLUTION TAKES ROOT

My patient Carolyn knew that her husband needed a trip to the dentist. But she had no idea how badly he needed it. She didn't know that a trip to the dentist could spell the difference between her husband's life and death.

Until recently, Carolyn hadn't been in great health either. But a few months earlier, she'd taken stock and decided to turn things around. She was at the top of her career, working as the editor for a nationally prestigious magazine. She had three brilliant children whom she was shipping off to college. And she was married to the best man she knew, a man who had been by her side since high school. She didn't want to lose all of that to poor health.

She had also written at least a dozen stories about the African American community's struggle with obesity, diabetes, and heart disease. Source after source had told her how important it is for black Americans to develop a culture of proactive health care. And yet she, herself, had not been to a dentist or doctor in years. It was time to start leading by example.

From where I sat, it was incredible to watch this woman transform her health. Over the course of a year, we worked together to get her mouth and body in tip-top shape. And every time she came into the office, I could see that she was fitter and more energetic than the last time. Somehow, the healthier she got, the more she enjoyed her work and appreciated the people in her life. Soon, her focus shifted from her own health to the health of her loved ones. So that one day she asked me whether I could give her next appointment to her husband instead.

She explained that he hadn't been to a doctor or dentist in years—that he was a sweet, gentle man who didn't like doctors poking and prodding or of dentists drilling and needling. "He says that his gums bleed on their own, and she was very concerned about the odor in his mouth," she concluded.

"That's not good," I said. "Bleeding gums usually means gum disease."

"I know. That's why I'd like you to see him."

So we made an appointment, and a week later, I had Carolyn and her husband sitting in my exam room.

Ken was exactly as Carolyn had described him—a sweet, soft-spoken man. I could see at once that he and Carolyn were meant for each other. But, as soon as I got a look inside his mouth, I realized that their marriage was at risk.

Ken reported that he felt fine, and he certainly looked lively. But his gums told a different story—one of inflammation and disease. We took his blood pressure as we routinely do on our patients and discovered that it was 200/105. That's what we call "hypertensive crisis." It meant that Ken could have an aneurysm, a stroke, or a heart attack at any moment.

"You need to get to an emergency room," I said. "I cannot treat you until your blood pressure is under control." Undiagnosed high blood pressure/hypertension is rampant in communities of color. If

I had a nickel for every time I diagnosed high blood pressure in our office ... you know how the saying goes. People visit their dentist more routinely than they even go to see the physician. The dentist becomes one of your most important primary health care providers because of that.

I explained what I had just discovered and gave Carolyn and Ken directions to the ER a few blocks away. Ken didn't seem too concerned as he left, but Carolyn hung back, looking terrified.

"Everything's going to be fine," I said. "Just get him to a hospital now."

I hugged her and she left.

It would be a year before I heard from Carolyn again.

As it turned out, Ken didn't make it to the emergency room that day. He said he didn't like doctors—that he'd give it a week and see how he felt. However, shortly thereafter, he'd had a stroke.

FROM TREAT IT AND BEAT IT TO TRANSFORMATIVE HEALTH

I've spent many years studying the connection between a healthy mouth and a long, healthy life. Oral health is not tangential—though some people have spent their entire lives ingesting that lie. What's happening in your mouth is an excellent indicator of what's happening in the rest of your body, providing a holistic snapshot of your overall health.

The problem is, many of today's practitioners aren't interested in holistic snapshots. They're fixers, highly skilled at what I call "treat it and beat it." They want to treat the current symptoms so they can beat the disease. And while I'm all for beating disease, that approach leaves something to be desired.

To understand where this attitude came from—and why it persists—we need to first understand the "growing pains" health care has gone through since the dawn of time. I want to introduce you to Dr. Chip Whitney, a pioneer in the field of transformative health, whose wisdom has had a powerful impact on my own complete health practice. It was Dr. Whitney who introduced me to the three eras of health identified by Dr. Lester Breslow in the American Journal of Public Health.

The first era started at the beginning of humankind. From the shamans and medicine men, early practitioners were literally and figuratively wandering around in the dark. Health providers didn't have a lot of tools, and the tools they did have often yielded results opposite from the ones they'd intended. Take, for example, the doctors who leeched sick people, believing their "bad blood" was at fault—and inadvertently killed their patients, who died from blood loss.

In the early days of human history, the focus was on battling infectious diseases. These diseases killed people in staggering numbers. The bubonic plague that swept through Europe in the fourteenth century—nicknamed the "Black Death"—killed an estimated fifty million men, women, and children: somewhere between 25 and 60 percent of the European population.

In light of statistics like that, no wonder the first era of health care was about survival. Infectious diseases were claiming millions of lives, so the only thing that mattered was trying to stop them through whatever means possible.

Now fast-forward a few hundred years. By the early 1900s, medicine had made significant advances. As public health trends improved, doctors and researchers had access to new tools and treatments. They developed antibiotics, which transformed the healthcare landscape forever.

In 1956, Elvis Presley posed publicly for his polio vaccination. This came at a time when tens of thousands of children were dying from polio, and those who weren't killed were often permanently paralyzed. Elvis's "plug" was highly effective: even though the vaccine had not yet been thoroughly tested, parents lined up to have their children inoculated.

Suddenly a world that had been shrouded in darkness was exposed to the light—and the second era of health care began.

If the first era was about battling infectious diseases, the second era was about combatting chronic diseases. In the latter half of the twentieth century, medicine advanced at an astonishing rate. Doctors began to identify and treat cancers. Surgery went from being a risky endeavor with terrifying instruments and a high mortality rate to a procedure that saved countless lives. Heart surgeons and brain surgeons undertook formidable challenges—and met them with flying colors. Over the last fifty years, the number of technology, medicine, and treatment options introduced has been revolutionary.

But how does that explain people like Cara Wells? How did a seemingly healthy thirty-six-year-old woman suffer a heart attack that nearly ended her life?

The answer is simple. The second era of health care, as wonderful as it is, is still fundamentally flawed. The mind-set of every physician in this country is "find the disease and fix it." In other words, "treat it and beat it." It is reactionary, not proactive. It treats the patient as an amalgam of symptoms and complaints, not a unique, complex human being who needs health care, not just sick care.

The third era of health care is about mind-set. We need a new mind-set among all health professions to help our patients create health, not just react to disease. The creation of health is not just about feeling OK today. It's about feeling great tomorrow—and all the tomorrows after that.

Our goal is to take a person who is not yet sick—who may not even have developed a problem—and prevent him or her from ever going down a path that will create illness.

Our main focus is simple yet powerful: we create health.

And who's at the cutting edge of this new third era?

We are. Your friendly neighborhood dentists.

IT'S ALL CONNECTED

I'm going to tell you something you might not want to hear.
Cara Wells could be anyone.
She could even be you.

In the human body, nothing happens in a vacuum. Everything is interconnected. But it is only now, in this third era of health care, that we are beginning to understand how and why.

You might be doing everything right: exercising, eating well, going in for your yearly checkups. If that's the case, more power to you. But if your dentist isn't lasering in on your oral health to look at the bigger picture, he or she is doing you a grave disservice, one that could mean the difference between life and death.

For years, dentistry has been associated with pain, both financial and physical. If that's the way you feel about going to see the dentist, I understand completely. Why would you willingly engage in something that only causes you pain? Only an idiot would sign up for that! I know exactly where you're coming from.

But I have good news for you. When you start thinking about dentistry in the context of complete health, it transforms from a place of pain and dread to a place of empowerment, where you, the patient, get to play an active role in your own care. Every day I partner with my patients in ways that are exciting, transformative, and even fun. Once you embrace the mouth as the gateway to complete health, great things can happen.

When I see a patient in my practice, my goal is not to drill, fill, and bill. I'm far more interested in the bigger picture of my patient's overall health.

That's why I use a process I like to call projection diagnostics. Projection diagnostics is a fancy term for a straightforward concept. I'm trying to project the patient's future health path by using diagnostic testing technologies, such as blood and urine tests. Based on the results of those tests, I like to project their future health path based on the results we find.

If a patient is on a bad health path, they can typically see where their problems lie, and we can course correct. The trickier patients are the ones like Cara Wells, people who seem to be healthy... but underneath the surface, there's something more serious going on.

When Cara first came to see me, I was determined to figure out why she had suffered from a heart attack. So I took off my white coat and donned my detective hat, ready to solve the mystery.

Cara was not at high risk for vascular disease. She was young, fit, and healthy. But I knew there must be something inflammatory going on because heart attacks are caused by inflammation, and the inflammation that led to the heart attack had to come from somewhere.

We used the process of elimination. Cara didn't have a sprained ankle. She had no open wound. So where was the inflammation coming from?

What she did have was a sore tooth.

I kept digging. I sent her to an endodontist who performed a root canal. What the endodontist discovered was that the tooth was badly infected. The bacteria from the infection likely entered her bloodstream and elicited an inflammatory reaction wherever they landed, including vulnerable coronary arteries, creating the ideal conditions for a heart attack.

That's right: a tooth infection drove Cara's vascular risk. What she thought of as a minor nuisance—a sore tooth, something a couple of ibuprofens could fix—had nearly ended her life and robbed her children of their mother.

THE MOUTH IS THE GATEWAY

America is the wealthiest nation in the world, yet we are one of the unhealthiest. If that surprises you, I understand. Until I shifted my focus to complete health, I didn't know all the depressing statistics—and I certainly didn't know how to change them. But there is evidence-based science to support the oral-systemic connection.

The mouth is the gateway to the body. It has key physiological functions that make it essential to our health and well-being; we eat with our mouths, we breathe through our mouths, and we kiss with our mouths. We have immunity through our mouths, and our oral health can even determine things like social status and hireability. If your teeth are badly decayed or missing entirely, you probably aren't going to get that front-row job.

For years doctors have overlooked the connection between what happens in a person's mouth and what happens in the rest of his or her body. The third era of health care requires a seismic shift. The better we understand—and care for—our oral cavity, the better chance we have of living a long, healthy life.

In this book, we're going to examine the mouth as a gateway to overall health. When bacteria from the oral cavity enter our bloodstream and spray everywhere, our body responds with inflammation, which sparks an inflammatory cascade. This cascade can lead to cardiovascular disease, dementia, cancers, sleep apnea, obesity, diabetes, and pregnancy complications—all of which we'll talk about in depth.

For each of these diseases, we'll look at the role your oral health plays, and explain how to identify—and treat—early warning signs. Every chapter includes sections titled "The Mouth-Body Connection" and "What Can You Do About It?" This is where I'll share specific treatment options and ways to predict and prevent serious disease so that you never find yourself in a situation like Cara Wells, facing a sudden heart attack with no idea why.

I don't want you to feel frightened and daunted after reading this book. I want you to feel empowered. My goal is to arm you with both the tools and the strategies you need to make informed decisions about your mouth, your health, and your life.

In the pages that follow, I'll introduce you to experts and practitioners who have studied chronic disease extensively and understand the crucial role of oral health. These doctors, nurses, and researchers are paving the way for a new kind of health care. They have not only revolutionized the way I run my practice; they are also leading the charge for Complete Health Dentistry® around the world.

You are standing at the precipice of the third era. Together, we have the power to transform health care in our world, our country, and our individual lives. True "health-care reform" isn't political. It's about treating the whole person and taking a long view, rather than slapping on a Band-Aid as a temporary solution.

It isn't about treating and beating.

It isn't about drilling and filling.

It isn't even about dentistry.

It's about you and your health. I want to ensure that you are happy and healthy for many years to come.

In order to do that, we have to talk about the original offender: the root cause of all the diseases we'll be discussing in this book.

I'm talking about the silent assassin that nearly ended Cara Wells's life at thirty-six years old.

Inflammation.

CHAPTER 3

INFLAMMATION: THE SILENT KILLER

I want you to imagine a beautiful antique car in an auto show. The paint is candy-apple red and polished to a fine sheen. The interior is flawless. The owner took very good care of his prized possession, so there's not a spot of rust on it—not even when you pop the hood. The car has impeccable maintenance records, and all these years later, if you turn the keys in the ignition, the engine still purrs.

Unfortunately, we human beings are rarely so well maintained.

Maybe you've had to face one or more diseases in your life. Maybe you haven't. But either way, you are rusting. That's just part of life on Earth. The scientific term for "rusting" is oxidation, which leads to inflammation, which leads to a host of nasty diseases that range from unpleasant to fatal.

We all live in a state of chronic inflammation. That's the basis for every single disease—cardiovascular disease, dementia, cancers, and other chronic ailments. In the last chapter, I talked about the inflammatory cascade. But since the word "inflammation" can feel esoteric and hard to quantify, I like to explain it in more concrete terms.

Let's say you're chopping vegetables in the kitchen. Your hand slips and you nick your finger with the knife. Nothing major—no need for a trip to the emergency room—but it stings, so you hold it under the faucet for a few minutes until it stops bleeding. Then you make an impromptu tourniquet out of a paper towel and go back to chopping vegetables for dinner.

For you, the cut is over.

For your body, it's only just begun.

Your skin serves as a barrier between the inside of your body and the harmful bacteria lurking on the outside: pathogens like bacteria, viruses, and other microorganisms. But now there's a break in the skin, providing a way for pathogens to enter your body. Once bacteria sneaks in through the cut, it can infect the wound.

Now, your body doesn't throw in the towel at the first glimpse of bacteria. On the contrary: when tissue is injured or infected, the body mounts a solid defense, releasing chemicals that trigger an inflammatory response to kill the invaders.

You might be thinking, Great, my body's a fighter! And that's true—at least initially. Your body ignites its inflammatory response to solve the problem and resolve the cut, and for a day or two, your fingertip gets red and puffy and feels sore. A week later, once the body has fought the bacteria and won, your finger is as good as new.

But when the triggers of inflammation never stop, our natural functioning can go haywire. Sometimes, when our bodies fight back, they don't know when to stop. This is chronic inflammation, which drives chronic disease.

THE WAR YOU DIDN'T KNOW YOU WERE FIGHTING

Let's talk about bacteria for a moment. These are microscopic organisms, and there are a lot of them. The global human population is currently around 7.6 billion, and saliva in the volume of a single nickel, you'll find 8 billion bacteria. That's right: one nickel yields more microscopic organisms than there are people on planet Earth.

There are 13 trillion bacteria in your intestines alone—so many that I've heard doctors describe them as an organ system in and of themselves. There are good bacteria and bad bacteria. When the delicate balance of the microbiome of your intestine gets out of whack and the bad outcompetes the good, it can lead to disease.

And then there's your mouth.

As we've established, the mouth is the gateway to the body. Unfortunately for your body, your mouth hosts billions of bacteria. Your tongue, teeth, and gums are bathing in bacteria at this very moment. Try not to think about that the next time you kiss your spouse!

Unfortunately for you, these pathogens get along fantastically with one another, so they stick together and multiply. Eventually, they form a colony, and after long enough, that colony creates a thick layer of plaque. Think of plaque like very bad house guests: they make your life a living nightmare . . . then stay forever.

If you've ever been to a dentist (and I hope you have), you've heard of plaque. But it's kind of like hearing the safety instructions on an airplane: after a while we've heard the words so many times, they no longer have any meaning.

Here's what you need to know about plaque: it spreads.

And I don't mean spreads in the way syrup oozes slowly over your pancakes. Plaque spreads like wildfire, taking over your mouth, teeth, tongue, cheeks—anywhere it can reach. If it can find an opening in your mouth that takes it directly to your bloodstream, all the better. The ravenous bacteria will happily stalk the rest of your body, wreaking havoc wherever and however they can.

But your body is wise to plaque's game. It prepares a counter-attack, waging war by firing inflammatory bullets on these foreign organisms—which in turn makes the plaque fight higher. Like any high school football team, the bacteria know the best defense is a good offense, so it launches barriers of resistance against the inflammatory attack.

In other words, there's a microscopic war raging inside you—and you have no idea.

You have a chronic inflammatory bacterial condition in your mouth. Chronic means your body never turns off the process of inflammation. It's like cutting your finger over and over and over again. The body is beleaguered by the constant assault of bacteria without an opportunity to resolve it, so the inflammatory response never powers down. What happens then?

You get sick.

THE DEADLY DANCE

As a part of his research on complete health transformation, Dr. Chip Whitney talks about three kinds of "body pollution" that lead to disease. Just like there is pollution in the air, pollution in the body drives people down certain chronic-disease paths. For Dr. Whitney the three main pollutants are oxidative stress, free radicals, and—you guessed it—inflammation.

At this point you may be thinking, I'm strong and healthy. I've never had a serious health problem or disease. Who's to say my body won't be able to fight off bacteria without causing chronic inflammation?

In a perfect world, your body would do just that. But this isn't a perfect world. If the cause of inflammation never stops, inflammation never turns off. The reality is that our bodies get worn down over time. We rust.

Some of the root causes of body pollution are minimally under our control. Take, for example, genetics and family history. We all have genetic predispositions to certain diseases, whether we like it or not. Then there's gut dysbiosis, where once again bad bacteria begin to dominate the good bacteria and throw everything out of balance. Insulin resistance, sleep apnea, high visceral (belly) fat—these are some of the root causes of pollution, and pollution is the root cause of disease.

It's important to note here that not all diseases are alike. In the last chapter, we talked about the bubonic plague, which we now know was caused by a single bacterium. Many illnesses can be traced back to one bacterium, including those that didn't cause sweeping epidemics, such as strep throat or pneumonia.

What I'm talking about is not a single bacterium. I'm talking about the massive hordes of bacteria that build up in the mouth and lower intestines and are dangerous because of quantity, not quality. Just one of them isn't going to cause a problem, but together they drive the infection. En masse, they steal into the bloodstream, triggering inflammation that can be transmitted to other organs.

Chronic inflammation is the root cause of almost all chronic disease. But there's one root cause of inflammation we haven't touched on. I saved the best for last.

Periodontal disease, a.k.a. gum disease.

As a dentist, I see a lot of gum disease. I have a front-row seat to inflammation in the tissues of the mouth. It starts as gingivitis, when your gums become swollen and red and may even bleed. As the disease progresses into full-blown periodontitis, the gums can pull away from the tooth, leading to bone loss and lost teeth.

Do you see how everything is connected? It all begins with bacteria, which causes periodontal disease. The pathogens trigger the body's inflammatory response, which in turn leads to inflammation in the mouth as the body tries to fight back. The mouth is the body's gateway, so the bacteria get into the bloodstream and spray everywhere, landing in the organs, the brain, and the arteries along the way, driving the same inflammation in those distant sites that is already present in the oral cavity.

And that, my friends, is a delicate, deadly dance that drives chronic disease.

THE THREE WAR ZONES

In the following chapters, we'll take a closer look at the three most worrisome diseases that result from inflammation. We'll start with cardiovascular disease, which covers heart attacks and strokes. A stroke is exactly the same as a heart attack, only it's a brain attack instead: same process, different location.

Then we'll talk about dementia. After that, we'll discuss various cancers, including colorectal, pancreatic, and esophageal. We'll also look at the interplay between inflammation and sleep apnea, obesity, diabetes, and pregnancy complications.

Here's my promise to you: this book is not all doom and gloom. There are ways to transform your health before you ever get sick.

That's why every chapter concludes with the answer to one simple question: "What Can You Do About It?" For each disease, I will share treatment options and other helpful resources. I want to show you how to change the path you're on before you end up at a destination you never want to visit.

The first step is to educate ourselves. If we don't know what we're looking for, we won't know how to fight it.

I'm a dentist, so I see all kinds of things in my practice. One thing that continues to amaze me is how many of my new patients tell me their gums bleed when they brush their teeth. "Just a little," they say. "Nothing major."

I want you to think about this for a moment. The total area of your gums is about the size of the palm of your hand. If you looked at the palm of your hand and saw an open wound, would you do something about it? Or would you continue to let it bleed?

Bleeding gums means there's an infection. Something is definitely wrong. But many people don't see it that way. They just spit a little blood and toothpaste into their bathroom sink in the morning and go on with their day.

The problem is, the mouth is only the beginning. Periodontal disease doesn't stop in your gums. Inflammation in the gums allows bacteria to spew into other parts of the body. Your organs. Your brain. Your heart.

Remember Cara Wells, the thirty-six-year-old who nearly died from a heart attack? She thought she was fine. Her risk-factor profile—based on her age, gender, genetic history, and general health and fitness—appeared to be low-risk. But she was harboring silent vascular disease. The inflammation from her mouth had traveled through her arteries, causing a blockage of blood flow to her heart.

This leads me to the question we've all been dying to ask: Was there anything Cara could have done to prevent it?

STRAIGHT TO THE HEART

At the beginning of this chapter, I asked you to imagine a mint-condition antique car at an auto show. Now I want you to envision yourself at ninety years old. What do you see? Do you see a polished antique automobile with an engine that still purrs? Or do you see a rusty, old mess when you pop the hood?

If you want to be healthy and happy at ninety, you need a healthy body and a healthy brain. You should be able to be as independent and active as you want to be. To get there, you need a strategy.

Most people don't have a strategy. We have plenty of strategies about our careers, finances, professional achievements, friendships, and even romantic relationships. But when we think about creating health, we tend to think in terms of losing weight, exercising, and eating well. That's it.

Those are tools to creating health, not strategies. At the heart of any good health strategy is identifying early disease. That's essential, because it is chronic disease that can steal life span from even the healthiest of individuals.

Identifying early disease can be challenging, especially when that disease is asymptomatic—as it usually is. Most of us do this in some form or another already: we schedule mammograms to screen for breast cancer, colonoscopies to screen for colon cancer, etc. Luckily for us, twenty-first-century technology is rapidly evolving, increasing our ability to identify disease at an early, treatable state.

The problem is that many diseases are untreatable once discovered.

So what do we do?

The answer is simple: we have to prevent the untreatable disease. We have to make the impossible possible. And the way to do that is by connecting the dots. We can prevent disease by reverse-engineering our way back to the inflammation that causes it in the first place.

The best way to start, of course, is to go straight to the heart.

CHAPTER 4

THE HEART OF THE MATTER

If I asked you to tell me the number one killer in this country, what would you say?

Car accidents?

Cancer?

The answer—which you've probably guessed from the chapter title—is heart disease.

Cardiovascular disease is the leading cause of death and disability for both men and women in the United States. Here's another statistic that will blow your mind: recent research has found that oral infections can trigger up to 50 percent or more of acute heart attacks!

That number is staggering, and it means Cara Wells is far from unique. The current cost of cardiovascular disease to our health-care system is about $518 billion. And guess what?

I believe it's preventable.

Prevention starts in the dentist's chair. But before we look at the link between a healthy mouth and a healthy heart, we have to understand how cardiovascular disease works—and why it's so dangerous.

OUT, DAMNED CLOT!

Cardiovascular disease is the umbrella term for a number of different events in the body, including:

- Aneurysm
- Angina
- Atherosclerosis
- Cerebrovascular accident (stroke)
- Cerebrovascular disease
- Congestive heart failure
- Coronary artery disease
- Electrical malfunctions like atrial fibrillation
- Myocardial infarction (heart attack)
- Peripheral vascular disease
- Valve diseases

In the last chapter we talked about plaque, the nightmare house guest nobody would ever want. The buildup of plaque causes the arteries (the blood vessels supplying oxygen to the heart) to narrow, making it harder for blood to flow. If someone is harboring silent plaque in his or her body, and the plaque ruptures like a volcano in the inner lining of the artery, it's bad news all around. That is a heart attack. If it occurs in the carotid artery in our neck, it causes a stroke or TIA (transient ischemic attack).

Remember how our bodies are trying so hard to protect us? When plaque ruptures the wall of an artery, our body says, "We better heal that injury!" In the same way a scab forms over the wound when a kid skins his or her knee, your body automatically sends a clotting cascade to heal the rupture of the artery wall.

If you shiver at the word "clotting," you should. A heart attack occurs when the blood flow to a part of the heart is blocked by a blood clot. If the clot cuts off the blood flow completely, the part of the heart muscle supplied by that artery begins to die.

This event usually occurs in a small blockage. Eighty-six percent of heart attacks occur from the rupture of a plaque so small that it would not have resulted in an abnormal stress test. Some of you may remember the ABC news anchorman Tim Russert. Tim had a completely normal stress test in April 2008. He died of a heart attack in June 2008. It was not that he had a bad doctor or a bad test; he just had a small plaque that did not show up during testing. A stress test is simply not an effective screening test.

In an ischemic stroke—which accounts for about 85 percent of strokes—the process is exactly the same; it just happens in a different location. The word ischemic comes from the Greek iskhaimos, or "stopping of blood." If the blood clot blocks blood flow in the heart, we call it a heart attack. If it floats from the carotid artery in the neck and lands in the brain, we call it a stroke. When the blood supply to a part of the brain is shut off, brain cells will die, impeding normal functions such as walking or talking.

Some of us are genetically predisposed to heart disease, and we can't change the genes we inherited. But there is one place where we can exercise a great deal of control.

You guessed it.

Our mouths.

THE MOUTH-ARTERY CONNECTION

As usual, the culprit is inflammation.

When oral bacteria enter the bloodstream and reach arteries, these arteries can incur the body's inflammatory wrath. The same inflammatory response that causes bleeding gums will occur in the walls of a vulnerable artery. Inflammation may cause the artery to rupture, then form a clot as the natural effort to heal the rupture, and, as you know, that can result in a heart attack or stroke.

There's a good deal of hard science on the link between oral health and heart disease. Studies published in prominent medical journals like Circulation, Journal of the American Heart Association, and The Lancet have shown the connection between infection in the mouth and cerebrovascular and cardiovascular disease. Major universities and medical institutions like the Cleveland Clinic are already changing their standard of care to incorporate the oral-systemic associations that research has uncovered.

Take, for example, the study done on 1,163 men, showing the oral bacterium Porphyromonas gingivalis to be associated with coronary heart disease (CHD). The same scientists went back and performed an even larger study of 6,950 subjects, providing serological evidence that an infection caused by major periodontal pathogens increased the risk of future stroke. Several years later, the National Institute of Health supported a third study in which researchers detected invasive periodontal pathogens at the sites of atherosclerotic disease. Bacterial presence in the artery wall was actually demonstrated through DNA technology.

In other words: a significant contributor to the plaque that built up in the walls of the patient's arteries had originated in his mouth!

Further investigative work needs to be performed, as is always the case with evidence-based research. But these studies—and numerous others—have established an unequivocal link. Now that we understand this important contributor to cardiovascular disease, we're able to develop novel therapies for treating it.

Of course, there will always be naysayers. In a recent guest editorial to the Journal of the American Dental Association, Bruce L. Pihlstrom called into the question the oral-systemic link, claiming, "There remains a need for more convincing and higher quality evidence that oral health care actually has a measurable impact on specific systemic diseases before it can be claimed that attaining good oral health can prevent systemic diseases or conditions."

The response from the American Academy for Oral Systemic Health was swift and mighty. The AAOSH board wrote a position paper in which they called out the JADA for their myopic, old-school thinking and failure to see the bigger picture.

"A little over a decade ago," the paper states, "we had no idea that the complexity of periodontal disease was enough to negatively influence glycemic control or cardiovascular health. But it is a disservice to unknowing patients when practitioners neglect the mounting associations, causation, and level-A evidence that infection in the mouth significantly contributes to medical conditions like heart attacks, stroke, Alzheimer's disease, cancers, diabetes, pre-term births, and a host of other inflammatory conditions."

As my friends and colleagues at the AAOSH noted, "Change is never easy. But the evidence of a significant association between oral and systemic health is incontrovertible. We must not let the complexity of this association deter us from expanding the nature and scope of our care when it is so clearly warranted."

As Dr. Whitney points out in his 2012 editorial published in Dentistry Today, "There is absolutely no risk to optimal dental care and home oral hygiene . . . What is the repercussion if we assume oral bacteria do not contribute to vascular disease and we are wrong? We miss the opportunity to significantly impact the lives of millions of people on the path to suffer a cardiovascular event!"

WOMEN WITH HEALTHY HEARTS

I want to introduce you to Dr. Gina Pritchard, cardiovascular nurse practitioner and the founder and director of The Prevent Clinic. For Dr. Pritchard, heart attacks and strokes are not an inevitable part of life. She travels and speaks as an advocate for early detection and prevention of heart disease, educating people everywhere on the importance of heart health.

We often think of breast cancer as the biggest health concern for women. Most of us know a woman who has fought it, and we see the signature pink ribbons everywhere we look. The whole month of October is dedicated to breast cancer awareness, and for good reason: one in thirty women will die of breast cancer.

It may surprise you to hear that one in three women will die of cardiovascular disease.

The PR campaign for detecting cardiovascular disease could learn a thing or two from breast cancer, because if heart disease had the same name recognition, thousands of lives might be saved. And yet cardiovascular disease kills more men and women than all kinds of cancer combined.

Dr. Pritchard has found that many people think of cardiovascular disease as a "man's disease," which simply isn't true. Heart attacks happen to just as many women as men, though they happen on average ten years later.

Women also have a different set of risk factors to contend with. For example, polycystic ovary syndrome (PCOS) is a hormonal disorder common among women. PCOS is a genetically driven type of insulin resistance that also increases the risk of cardiovascular disease. If you are a woman with PCOS—or if you have a wife, sister, mother, or daughter with PCOS—early screening is all the more essential.

Because women often experience different symptoms of cardiovascular disease than men, it can sometimes be harder to detect. In the months before a heart attack, a woman might be unusually fatigued—which they could just as easily chalk up to a bad night of sleep. They might also experience indigestion, weak arms, a racing heart, or anxiety. While a man might complain of gripping chest pains during a heart attack, women can have subtler, less recognizable symptoms, such as nausea, pain or discomfort in the back, stomach, jaw, or neck, and shortness of breath. Because women are often unaware these symptoms might mean a heart attack or cardiovascular disease, they ignore the signs.

"I give a female twist to the complete health workup," Dr. Pritchard says. "Not just in the dental office, but the collaborative practice model where the dental community, dental team, and the medical team are working together in an integrated approach. We want to screen, appropriately diagnose, and then either treat existing cardiovascular disease—or prevent early-stage atherosclerosis from developing. We can prevent an event in the future for patients with or without existing cardiovascular disease.

Dr. Pritchard believes strongly in early-stage screening. She goes around the country championing the carotid intima-media thickness ultrasound, which is being performed in more and more dental offices—and rightly so. "I did my doctoral work on early screening," Pritchard says, "and it's something that I'm helping dentists, dental hygienists, MDs, DOs, and nurse practitioners with in offices all across the United States." She hopes to expand to other countries as Complete Health Dentistry® goes global.

Preventing cardiovascular disease is possible—but you won't know how to treat it if you don't know where to look.

WHAT CAN YOU DO ABOUT IT?

Here's the good news: unlike many other chronic medical conditions, cardiovascular disease is treatable and can be reversible, even after a long history of disease.

The first step is detection. As Dr. Gina Pritchard and Dr. Chip Whitney can attest, early screening could save your life. That vital journey might begin with a trip to the dentist—as long as your dentist is an advocate and practitioner of Complete Health Dentistry®.

I want to introduce you to Brad Bale, MD and Amy Doneen, MSN, ARNP, DNP. Ten years ago, when Dr. Bale and Dr. Doneen first started working together, they began to investigate the oral-systemic link. They learned that, although there are many pathologies that drive vascular events, oral health doesn't seem to get enough attention in the medical world. The more they looked into the data and literature, the more convinced they became that the same bacteria that cause periodontal disease cause heart attacks and ischemic strokes.

So why wasn't oral health getting enough credit? Because the medical and dental communities just did not understand. They decided to take matters into their own hands.

Together, the doctors founded the BaleDoneen Method® for preventing heart attacks, strokes, and Type 2 diabetes. Now they teach physicians, dentists, and other health-care providers around the world their method for early detection and treatment.

For Dr. Bale and Dr. Doneen, a critical component of early detection and treatment is simple: Go to the dentist. Get your teeth and gums evaluated regularly, and accept the recommended treatment plan when you need to—not just so you can have pretty teeth, but because it might save your life.

"Periodontal disease is extremely prevalent," says Dr. Bale. "Once you're thirty years of age, there's a 50 percent chance you have it. Once you're sixty-five, there's an 80 percent chance. If you don't want to have a heart attack or stroke, you need to maintain a healthy mouth, be evaluated thoroughly for periodontal disease, and if it's present, eradicate it."

Dr. Bale and Dr. Doneen are so confident in their work that they actually guarantee it: since 2008, they have offered all patients treated at their clinics—the Heart Attack & Stroke Prevention Center in Spokane, Washington, and the Heart Attack, Stroke and Diabetes Center at the Grace Clinic in Lubbock, Texas—a written guarantee stating that if the patient suffers a heart attack or stroke while under their care, the doctors will refund 100 percent of the fees paid during the year.

"We get extremely high-risk patients," says Dr. Bale, "which is fine. I like a challenging patient, and I do believe you can shut down the disease process in anybody."

Dr. Bale and Dr. Doneen have worked tirelessly to synthesize all the data and develop the BaleDoneen Method® because they truly believe that heart attacks and strokes are preventable. You can read more about their work at baledoneen.com.

In addition to staying on top of your periodontal care, here are some other ways to minimize your risk of having a stroke or heart attack:

- Control high blood pressure (hypertension).
- Identify inflammatory cholesterol and prediabetes early.
- Follow good oral-health maintenance practices that promote healthy gums and teeth.
- Quit tobacco use.
- Eliminate inflammatory visceral (belly) fat.
- Eat a diet rich in fruits and vegetables.
- Exercise regularly.
- Drink alcohol in moderation, if at all.
- Know your genetics.
- Establish and maintain gut health.

The following are some resources that might be helpful:

heart.org/HEARTORG/Caregiver
periodontal.com
news-medical.net
perio.org/consumer/mbc.heart
oralsystemiclink.net
aaosh.org/
RHSLiveWell.com

WHAT'S NEXT?

Now that we've talked about heart health, it's time to move onward and upward. Because your mouth doesn't only tell us a lot about your cardiovascular health; it also tells us all about your brain.

CHAPTER 5

DON'T FORGET

Jeffrey Jameson's pearly whites might not have been pearly white anymore, but his was still the most beautiful smile I'd ever seen.

Back in 2002, when my son was turning six years old, he got a brand spanking new shiny red bike for his birthday. The way my son smiled that day—that's how Jeffrey smiled.

Jeffrey said he was smiling because this was the first time he could remember meeting an African American dentist, and a female. But I took that with a grain of salt: Jeffrey hadn't been to the dentist in a decade, and he couldn't remember much of anything these days.

His daughter, Sheila, was about fifty years old and explained that as her father aged, his health, sleep, and memory had begun dropping off. She'd been caring for him ever since. This morning, they were getting his teeth looked at, and in the afternoon, they'd be getting him a physical.

When I heard that he wasn't sleeping well—only about four or five hours a night—I decided to make a sleep appliance for Jeffrey. And given his poor health, I suggested that we take a cone beam x-ray first, prior to making the appliance.

"What're you expecting to find?" Sheila asked.

"Hopefully nothing," I said.

Sheila looked nervous. "It's just the time," she said. "We've got this doctor's appointment we have to get to."

I explained that I could take the x-rays and email the results once the images developed. Sheila agreed. So we took the x-rays and sent the Jamesons on their way.

But when we got the results back an hour later, I didn't email Sheila. I called her instead. And I was very serious.

The call went to Sheila's voicemail, so I hung up and redialed. Voicemail. Redial. Voicemail. Redial. And then I heard those three words I'd been praying for.

"This is Sheila."

I took a deep breath and said, "We found something."

Fortunately, I had caught her while she was still at the doctor's office. Sheila handed the phone over to the doctor, and we talked through the results of the x-ray. The scan had revealed a blockage in Jeffrey's carotid artery. It was cutting off the flow of oxygen to his brain. Mr. Jameson was a ticking time bomb—he could have a stroke at any moment.

As soon as the doctor heard that, she just said "Thanks," and hung up. There was no time to talk. She had to get Jeffrey into an operating room as quick as she could.

A little while later, I learned that the doctors had performed a stenting procedure, placing a metal tube inside the artery, which would open it up and restore the flow of oxygen.

The discovery we made explained Jeffrey's memory loss. Jeffrey wasn't just getting old. The blockage in his carotid artery had been slowly suffocating his brain, killing off cells and prompting the onset of dementia. It was possible that the stenting procedure might restore some of Jeffrey's memory, but probably not most of it. Given how long it had been since the last time Jeffrey got looked at, chances were that his brain had been oxygen-deprived for years. The dementia would probably be permanent.

If you're one of the lucky few whose life has never been touched by Alzheimer's disease, chances are your luck won't last forever. An estimated 5.7 million Americans live with Alzheimer's disease (AD)—also known as senile dementia of the Alzheimer type (SDAT)—and that number is expected to grow to 15 million by 2060.

Put another way, someone in the United States develops AD every sixty-five seconds. By the middle of this century, someone in the US will develop the disease every thirty-three seconds.

The face of Alzheimer's may not be what you think. Early-onset AD is becoming more prevalent, so that while the vast majority of people facing the disease are still over sixty-five, some are younger. In 2018, approximately 200,000 individuals under age sixty-five had early-onset Alzheimer's disease.

Many of us fear we are headed toward a future of forgetting the people we love—especially those of us who've watched friends and family members decimated by this cruel, devastating disease. I won't lie to you: the statistics aren't encouraging. According to the Alzheimer's Association, "Alzheimer's disease is the only top-ten cause of death in the United States that cannot be prevented, cured, or even slowed." This is arguably the most important disease Dr. Whitney refers to when he says we must prevent the untreatable.

The good news is: times are changing. There are an increasing number of studies suggesting what causes it. The more we learn about AD, the better chance we have of learning how to take precautionary measures to help protect ourselves before it strikes.

Scientists and researchers have made—and continue to make—exciting new discoveries in the study of Alzheimer's disease that point to the link between AD and inflammation. The field of research is still young, and more studies are needed to yield conclusive results. But the research suggests that exposure to inflammation early in life can quadruple one's risk of developing Alzheimer's disease later on.

First, let's talk about what Alzheimer's is, what it isn't, and how this brutal disease has left scientists scratching their heads for a very long time.

IS ALZHEIMER'S THE SAME AS DEMENTIA?

You've probably heard "Alzheimer's disease" and "dementia" used interchangeably. The reason for this confusion may be your doctor's fault. The word Alzheimer's tends to evoke fear and panic, so some physicians will use the term dementia instead. They're not entirely wrong. Alzheimer's is one type of dementia. But they're not synonymous.

According to the National Institute of Neurological Disorders and Stroke (NINDS), dementia is "a group of symptoms caused by disorders that affect the brain. It is not a specific disease."

NINDS goes on to say, "People with dementia may not be able to think well enough to do normal activities, such as getting dressed or eating. They may lose their ability to solve problems or control their emotions. Their personalities may change. They may become agitated or see things that are not there."

If you find yourself thinking, Those symptoms sound like Alzheimer's symptoms, you are correct. There are several types of dementia, but Alzheimer's is the most common. AD is a neurodegenerative disorder defined by the Alzheimer's Foundation of America as "a progressive, degenerative disorder that attacks the brain's nerve cells, or neurons, resulting in loss of memory, loss of thinking and language skills, and behavioral changes."

Fun fact: AD was named after a German physician, Alois Alzheimer, who first described it in 1906. Sometimes I wonder how Alois would feel if he knew his name was known the whole world over, but associated with dread and fear. Maybe an incurable disease is not the way you want to be remembered.

As more and more nerve cells die, Alzheimer's disease leads to significant brain shrinkage. And since the brain runs so many of the body's operations, when your brain powers down, you power down too.

The symptoms of Alzheimer's can vary in severity and chronology. But the overall progress of the disease is fairly predictable. AD is terminal; on average, people live eight to ten years after diagnosis, though they can sometimes live up to twenty. In the later stages, autonomic functions like heart rate, breathing, digestion, and autoimmune response are affected.

While the disease is fatal, it's often secondary illnesses that cause death, everything from heart attacks to kidney failure to pneumonia. Advanced Alzheimer's patients are usually too frail, their immune systems too compromised, to fight off bacterial infections that a healthier person could survive.

ALZHEIMER'S AND INFLAMMATION: A STICKY BOND

There's a lot of debate about what causes Alzheimer's disease, and the various theories often get contentious. Most scientists will concede that Alzheimer's results from a combination of genetic, lifestyle, and environmental factors that affect the brain over decades.

One thing we can all agree on is that there is plaque in the brains of Alzheimer's patients. As a dentist, I obviously talk a lot about plaque. But whereas plaque in your mouth is made up of sticky deposits between your teeth, neurological plaques are abnormal clusters of protein fragments that gum up and block the functioning of brain cells. It's like what would happen if you spilled soda on your laptop: the sticky liquid would gum up the circuitry and ruin your computer. The plaque spreads through the cortex in a predictable pattern as the disease progresses.

Where the plaque comes from—and why it so viciously attacks the brain's nerve cells—remains something of a mystery. Despite the billions of dollars that have been invested to crack the case, scientists are still not certain.

"We have done absolutely nothing to change the course of the disease," says Dr. Garth Ehrlich, a professor at Drexel University College of Medicine. "Other chronic diseases, we have affected, because we understand what causes them. There is nothing new you can do for an Alzheimer's patient that you couldn't do twenty years ago."

Dr. Ehrlich isn't the only one who feels that the direction of Alzheimer's research needs to be rerouted. His colleague Dr. Herbert Allen, chairman of Drexel's Department of Dermatology, became fascinated by research showing a link between Alzheimer's and bacteria in the brain. He pored over the work done by Swiss researcher Judith Miklossy, who found two types of spirochetes—long, corkscrew-shaped bacteria—in the brains of more than 90 percent of Alzheimer's disease patients. Her research suggested that most of these spirochetes originated from the mouth. Miklossy's paper, published in

2011, was soon corroborated by other studies that found a connection between bacteria and dementia.

In 2016, Dr. Allen conducted his own study. He and his team of scientists investigated seven post-mortem brains of patients with Alzheimer's disease, comparing them to ten healthy brains. The results suggested that spirochetes in the brain could be creating "biofilms," films of bacteria that are slimy, glue-like, and incredibly resistant to antibiotics.

When he published the results of his study in the Journal of Neuroinfectious Diseases, Allen hypothesized that "spirochetes enter the brain during a dental procedure or after a person contracts Lyme, and then spin out a protective biofilm. The body's first responders try to clear the infection, but . . . the immune system ends up destroying the surrounding tissue."

According to Dr. Allen, the cause of Alzheimer's disease may be a body's own immune system mounting an inflammatory defense—one that could be triggered from a dental procedure or chronic inflammation of the gums.

Sound familiar?

Make no mistake: Dr. Allen's hypothesis is highly controversial. The traditional medical community loves to discredit researchers who find proof of a connection between dementia and oral health. Further research is certainly needed to confirm that spirochetal bacteria—or any bacteria—can trigger the inflammatory cascade that leads to Alzheimer's disease.

But as more research is done on the link between bacteria and Alzheimer's, I believe we'll see increasing evidence of the crucial importance of a healthy mouth. Spirochetes, the offending bacteria, are found in the oral cavity. That's a fact. And since spirochetal infection occurs years or even decades before dementia manifests, a patient could potentially prevent and eradicate Alzheimer's years before it began. Remember Dr. Whitney's comment, "What is the repercussion if we assume oral bacteria do not contribute to disease and we are wrong?" This applies to Alzheimer's disease too. We have an opportunity to prevent the untreatable.

WHAT CAN YOU DO ABOUT IT?

Since there are currently no medically sanctioned ways to prevent Alzheimer's disease, this is a tricky question. Since the research on neuroinflammation is new—though growing—we're still wandering in the dark.

But there is light at the end of the tunnel as scientists and researchers begin to illuminate the path. Dr. Dale Bredesen, a professor of neurology at the David Geffen School of Medicine at UCLA, recently launched a years-long study on ten patients with Alzheimer's dementia. The results of the study, published in the journal Aging, were landmark, the first to suggest that memory loss in patients may, in fact, be reversed. Bredesen used a complex, thirty-six-point therapeutic program that involved comprehensive diet changes, brain stimulation, exercise, sleep optimization, specific pharmaceuticals and vitamins, and multiple additional steps that affect brain chemistry.

For me, the results of Bredesen's work are encouraging. I believe an inflammatory burden early in life, as represented by chronic periodontal disease, could have severe consequences later as a contributing factor to Alzheimer's. If the link between inflammation and Alzheimer's disease is confirmed, researchers say it would add reducing inflammatory burden to the short list of preventable risk factors for Alzheimer's disease.

What does this mean for you?

It means go to your dentist regularly, accept the recommended treatment plan, and do everything in your power to combat inflammation when—or better yet, before—it strikes.

The following are some resources that might be helpful:

medicalnewstoday.com
mayoclinic.com/health/alzheimers-disease
ahaf.org/alzheimers/about/symptomsandstages
alz.org/alzheimers-dementia/what-is-alzheimers/
drbredesen.com/thebredesenprotocol

WHAT'S NEXT?

We've talked about cardiovascular health and brain health—how inflammation can lead to a heart attack and might even cause brain cells to die.

But what about other systems of the body? Does inflammation cause widespread health problems in organs like your colon or your lungs?

You bet it does. In the next chapter, I'll explain how.

CHAPTER 6

AN INFLAMED BODY IS A SICK BODY

The WWRL 1600 AM radio station has been serving New Yorkers since the 1920s. It's been Hungarian, Italian, French, Greek, and Polish. It's been Spanish, Ukrainian, Russian, and Scandinavian. In the years that I listened to it, WWRL primarily served the African American community and had a wonderful Caribbean following as well. People listened for talk shows, the politics, and in the evenings, there was a Latin and Caribbean community listened.

This was in the early 2000's, and the idea of writing a book still hadn't occurred to me. But I knew that I wanted to find some way to start talking about the importance of oral health care. I didn't want to be one of those dentists who holes themselves up in their office, treating only the patients who think to make appointments. I wanted to reach a broader population.

So I talked to some people, and they talked to some people, and we came up with a plan: every Sunday, I would spend an hour in

WWRL's Chelsea studio, monologuing about holistic approaches to health care.

One night, on my way out of the studio, I ran into a DJ named Marcus. Marcus's income relied on his ability to talk in a way that made you want to listen. Marcus was a heavy smoker. During his breaks he would find himself going outside in all types of weather for a smoke break before coming in and playing more music. When I asked him how long it had been since his last trip to the dentist, he just smiled. Marcus had been listening to my show, and he started asking questions about the connection between the mouth and the rest of the body. Soon thereafter, he decided to make an appointment in my office.

Within a few days, I had Marcus lying in the patient's chair under my overhead light. During patients' initial examinations, I obtain their medical history, and ask them about their diet, lifestyle, and other habits so I can get to know a bit more about my them, other than just the teeth. Marcus said he had a rather normal diet, and he exercised regularly, however, it was his pack a day cigarette habit that was very concerning to me.

"Open wide," I said. And he did. We proceeded with a thorough examination, starting outside the mouth and palpating the muscles of his head and neck. Afterwards, I proceeded to check the muscles inside his mouth, including his tongue, all the way to the back of his throat to the tonsils. Afterward, I checked his cheeks, the floor of the mouth, and then the teeth and gums. It was during the examination of the gums that I noticed this white and red lesion on the side of his gums towards his molars. I sat back, removed my gloves, and turned off the lamp.

"What's wrong?" he asked.

"I'm not sure," I said. "But you've got this lesion towards the back of your mouth that I want to biopsy. It needs further evaluation."

We did a brush biopsy of the lesion, which is a very simple test that we perform in our office when we see areas of concern. We will rub a little bristle-like brush over the lesion, and the sample is then sent to the laboratory where they look at the cells under a microscope to see if they are suspicious for cancer.

A week later, the tests came back positive for cancerous cells. Marcus had oral cancer. We then sent Marcus to an oral surgeon so that he could have further testing and treatment. Fortunately, we'd caught it early. Surgeons removed a bit of jaw bone and a few lymph nodes. And like that, the cancer was gone.

"I'm so glad we caught in time," Marcus said a few weeks later. "If I'd waited much longer to see someone, they might have had to remove the whole jaw. It'd be pretty impossible to DJ without your jaws."

"Marcus," I said, "if you'd waited much longer, you wouldn't be alive anymore."

Every sixty minutes, one person dies from oral cancer. That's one person every hour, twenty-four hours a day. Contrary to what many people think, it isn't relegated to people who smoke or chew tobacco; it affects people of all ages, nationalities, and walks of life. Oral cancer is one of the biggest killers in our country, but it's a silent epidemic. No one talks about it.

THE DREADED C-WORD

We all know someone who has won a battle against a cancer. We also all know someone who hasn't.

Cancer isn't choosy; it picks its victims regardless of age, race, sex, gender, and socioeconomic status. Even Steve Jobs, the man who created a veritable tech empire and had access to the best health care in the world, died of pancreatic cancer, proving that no amount of money or power can turn back time.

Like many of the diseases we've discussed in this book, there are varying theories about what causes cancer. Research has found a connection between some cancers and what happens in the oral cavity.

In 2015, a group of Korean scientists set out to study periodontitis, the most common chronic inflammatory condition in the mouth. They investigated Porphyromonas gingivalis, a major pathogen of chronic periodontitis, exploring the role it plays in oral cancer.

The results of their study were exciting—and revolutionary. The researchers found that P. gingivalis can indeed increase the aggressiveness of oral-cancer cells. When it comes to cancer of the mouth, periodontitis poses a serious bacterial risk.

Oral cancer isn't the only kind of cancer that is being studied by researchers as they continue to investigate the importance of a healthy mouth. Scientists have also proposed a link between oral health and esophageal, pancreatic, and colorectal cancer.

Colon cancer is cancer of the large intestine, the lower part of your digestive system; rectal cancer is cancer of the last several inches of the colon. Together, they are referred to as colorectal. Most cases begin as small, noncancerous (benign) clumps of cells called adenomatous polyps; in certain cases, some of these polyps become cancerous over time.

About 136,000 people in the United States are diagnosed with colorectal cancer each year, and of those, 50,300 are predicted to die from the disease. It is the third most commonly diagnosed cancer and the third leading cause of cancer death.

Two independent studies were recently published in the journal Cell Host & Microbe, one from Harvard and the other from Case Western Reserve University. In each study, scientists looked at a strain of mouth bacteria that causes gum disease to determine the role it played in colorectal cancer. The bacteria in question were Fusobacteria.

Fusobacteria starts off in the mouth and is frequently associated with gum disease. Earlier studies hadn't observed the bacteria within the actual tumors, which led researchers at Harvard to look at earlier stages of colon cancer to see if this discrepancy was merely an issue of timing.

Their hunch was correct: they found fresh evidence that Fusobacteria were intimately nestled within tumors of the colon. In other words, the bacteria from the oral cavity made their way to the colon, though researchers have not yet definitively proven if the bacteria move through the blood or the GI tract.

They didn't stop there. The Harvard researchers found that Fusobacteria elevated the generation of tumors in a mutant mouse strain prone to developing intestinal cancer. Infection with these microbes attracts a particular brand of immune cell—myeloid cells—which the researchers found stimulate the inflammatory responses that can cause cancer.

Inflammation was on the prowl again, this time, leading to colorectal cancer. The proof was in the colon.

BREATHE IN, BREATHE OUT

In this chapter we've talked about cancer, but there's another deadly disease that has been linked to oral health (or the lack thereof): lung disease.

Lung disease is another one of those umbrella terms with many diseases nested under it. It is technically any problem in the lungs that prevents them from working properly. Tens of millions of people suffer from lung disease in the US alone.

There are three main types of lung disease:

1. Airway diseases: These affect the tubes (airways) that carry oxygen and other gases into and out of the lungs.

2. Lung-tissue diseases: These affect the structure of the lung tissue.

3. Lung-circulation diseases: These affect the blood vessels in the lungs.

Many lung diseases involve a combination of these three types. Take, for example, chronic obstructive pulmonary disease (COPD), one of the most common lung diseases. COPD comes in two main forms: chronic bronchitis, which involves a long-term cough with mucus; and emphysema, which involves damage to the lungs over time. Smoking, genetics, and infections—including periodontal infections—are responsible for most lung diseases.

There is a fair amount of evidence linking pneumonia to oral health. Scientists have also done a good deal of research to show that good oral hygiene and frequent professional oral health care reduce the progression or occurrence of respiratory diseases among high-risk elderly living in nursing homes, especially those in intensive care units.

Similar studies have shown that lung function decreases with increasing periodontal attachment loss. In layman's terms: your lungs get worse the more the periodontal support around a tooth—the bone and tissue—has been destroyed.

All of this research lends credence to a potential association between periodontitis and chronic pulmonary diseases like COPD.

AND THAT'S NOT ALL

In this chapter we've barely scratched the surface of the different diseases in the body that have been linked to oral health. Additional studies have pointed to a link between inflammation and kidney disease, liver disease, and numerous others.

When I see patients in my practice, these are the kinds of things I'm looking for. I often think of my neighbor, who implored me to do for others what I did for her.

"I hope you encourage all of your patients to focus on prevention," she told me. "I shudder to think what might have happened if you hadn't been looking so carefully."

WHAT CAN YOU DO ABOUT IT?

As with all the diseases we've discussed in this book, there's no "tried and true" method to prevention. You can control and maintain your oral health and other aspects of your lifestyle, but, of course, there are some things you can't control, like your genetics.

Here's the thing: you can control inflammation, starting right in the dentist's chair. You can do everything in your power to prevent the inflammation that has been linked to cardiovascular disease; stroke; dementia and Alzheimer's disease; colorectal, pancreatic, and esophageal cancer; and diseases of the lungs, kidneys, and liver.

Yes, additional research is needed. That's how science works. Study by study, case by case, the tide begins to turn. But the writing is on the wall. In the field of oral-systemic health, the body of evidence continues to grow. No one disputes the destructive nature of chronic inflammation. If there is anything you can do to prevent, treat, and correct it, do it. DO IT NOW.

The following are some resources that might be helpful:

cancer.org
emedicinehealth.com
webmd.com
medicaldaily.com
nlm.nih/gov/medlineplus/ency/article/000066.htm
mayoclinic.com
webmd.com/lung/lung-diseases-overview

WHAT'S NEXT?

We've talked about a number of diseases that may be caused by the inflammation triggered by periodontal disease. Now we're going to change it up a bit and talk about some root causes of inflammation outside of the mouth, including obesity, diabetes, and a condition that strikes while you're sound asleep.

That's right: the root causes of disease don't rest, even when you are trying to.

Let's talk about sleep apnea and its stealthy assault.

CHAPTER 7

THE POWER OF A GOOD NIGHT'S SLEEP

When I moved to New York over twenty years ago, I only knew a few people. But New York is a great place to make friends. It seems that most people are from somewhere else and move to New York, New York, a city so nice, they named it twice. One of the first friends that I met was Ava. We had so much in common. We both came from the same city and had attended the same university—the list goes on. Ava and I went out for drinks once and we've been friends ever since.

Never have I ever met anyone with who is such a beautiful soul with her energy and her sense of play. An evening with her is an evening of nonstop laughter and nonstop movement. Just spend five minutes with her and you'll see what I mean: the woman is caring, lovable and fun.

To me, that restlessness is fun and charming. But Ava says that for her, it can sometimes be a burden. She feels like she can never relax.

"What do you mean?" I asked her once, a few months after we met.

"Well, for one thing," she said, "I'm basically incapable of sleeping."

As soon as the words were out of her mouth, a light bulb went off in my head. This wasn't the first time I'd heard Ava talk about sleeplessness. In fact, I'd been hearing about it since I'd known her. She'd forget her purse somewhere and say her brain was just tired. Or she'd reschedule a dinner because she was too tired to go out. We never got together before noon because Ava said she didn't like to socialize "half asleep." And I'd gotten more three-in-the-morning emails from her than I could count.

As soon as I put all of that together, I recommended that Ava come in for a sleep test.

She did, and a few days later, I found myself handing her a brochure on sleep apnea.

"You don't need to relax," I told Ava. "You need to breathe."

I want to introduce you to Dr. Michael Gelb, a dentist, author, speaker, and sleep specialist at the Gelb Center in New York City. Dr. Gelb specializes in TMJ, headaches, sleep disorders, and sleep apnea. He believes that 50 percent of the patients we dentists see in our practice on any given day may struggle with an undiagnosed airway problem. Not a sleep problem. Not a breathing problem. They have a narrowed airway—and they're paying a high price.

Over the years, Dr. Gelb has developed razor-sharp sensibilities. Within a few minutes of examining a patient and listening to them describe their symptoms, he can often tell whether or not they have an airway problem. It's why he launched the Gelb Center, which now maintains two offices dedicated to AirwayCentric® dentistry, oral/systemic wellness, and anti-inflammatory dentistry. Through his work, he has been able to transform countless lives and has developed the AirwayCentric® Guide (ACG) System for dentists and healthcare providers who wish to implement AirwayCentric® and Complete Health® practice. More on that later.

In this chapter, I want to share some of Dr. Gelb's wisdom with you. He believes that a clear, healthy, unobstructed airway is the hidden path to well-being—and so do I.

WHAT IS SLEEP APNEA?

Many of us are tired. Day in and day out, we go through our lives in a state of chronic exhaustion. We may go to bed late and get up early. We may have to be up before our kids every morning; we frantically get them ready for school at the same time we get ourselves ready for work. As a consequence of our overscheduled, overcommitted lives, no one's getting enough sleep.

We all know that when we are tired, we're not our best self. We're more susceptible to catching a cold or—heaven forbid—being laid flat on our back with a case of the flu. But not sleeping well isn't just a minor inconvenience. It can have serious, long-term effects on your health.

If you sleep three to four hours a night, you're going to be tired no matter what I do for you. Many of my patients dutifully get their seven to eight hours of sleep a night and still wake up heavy with fatigue. They can't figure out why they're so tired, and as we start to trace their symptoms back to the source, we realize something else is going on.

When you breathe, air travels down your throat through your windpipe. The narrowest part of that pathway is in the back of your throat. When you're awake, muscles keep that pathway relatively wide open. When you sleep, those muscles relax, allowing the opening to narrow. The air passing through this narrowed opening may create vibrations. These vibrations in your throat cause snoring.

Snoring is not necessarily indicative of a health issue. But for some people, the throat closes too much and not enough air can get through to the lungs. When this happens, the brain sends an alarm to open the airway—and you are briefly roused from sleep. Many times, this also wakes the person sleeping next to you.

The brain quickly reactivates the muscles that hold the throat open so air can get through again, and once all is free and clear, the brain goes back to sleep. The person lying next to you may remain awake much longer.

This disorder is called obstructive sleep apnea (OSA).

OSA is breathing interrupted by a physical block to airflow despite respiratory effort. Eighty-four percent of sleep apnea is OSA, making it the most common form. The other type of apnea, central sleep apnea (CSA), is breathing interrupted by a lack of respiratory effort. Complex or mixed sleep apnea is a combination of OSA and CSA.

All types of sleep apnea create abnormal pauses in breathing—or instances of abnormally low breathing—during sleep. Each pause can last from a few seconds up to whole minutes, and may occur five to thirty times (or more) an hour.

Have you ever been trying to watch a movie at home, but you keep getting interrupted? Maybe your child keeps running in to ask you questions, or your internet service keeps dropping, a colleague is bombarding you with text messages, or your dog keeps barking at people walking outside. Mine barks every time a dog is on the TV screen!

If you have to pause your movie five to thirty times in an hour, do you think you'll be able to hold on to the thread of the plot? I'm guessing not!

That's how it is when you have sleep apnea. Your body loses the thread of the plot—the plot being a restful night's sleep.

Symptoms of both OSA and CSA include daytime sleepiness and fatigue, snoring, restless sleep, and awakening with a dry mouth or sore throat. One in four patients with OSA suffer from nighttime teeth grinding, which can wear down the teeth and destroy the enamel.

It gets worse. Researchers have revealed that people with obstructive sleep apnea show tissue loss in brain regions that help store memory, linking OSA with memory loss. Sleep fragmentation leads to inflammation—and as we've established, inflammation can make you sick.

Despite the long list of symptoms, people who suffer from sleep apnea are rarely aware of having difficulty breathing, even upon waking. You might experience chipped teeth or reflux—little hints and clues leading to sleep apnea—but the disorder is usually only recognized by a partner or friend who has witnessed an episode. Like so many harmful diseases, you may have no idea you're sick. Sleep apnea robs you of your health and vitality—and like a midnight thief, it does so while you sleep.

So far in this book, we've talked about how inflammation is a key player—the central villain, you might say—in oral-systemic health. We've seen how it can drive cardiovascular disease, dementia, and cancer, and we know that bacteria in the gums and mouth can trigger an inflammatory cascade.

Dr. Gelb points to an additional cause; Gelb believes that airway/sleep disorders are the most prominent cause of systemic inflammation, as well as oxidative stress, endothelial dysfunction, and sympathetic overload. This is why he has dedicated his life's work to helping patients open their airways. If he can increase oxygenation to allow deep sleep, he can improve cardiovascular disease, cerebrovascular disease, diabetes, and even dementia and Alzheimer's disease. Oxygen can also help eradicate the microorganisms that exist in the mouth.

Dr. Gelb refers to those microorganisms as bad bugs.

"It is not by coincidence that the bad bugs in our mouth are anaerobic," he says, "meaning, they thrive in low-oxygen environments."

What that means is when we open the airway and increase systemic oxygen, it helps to reduce oral bacteria from the inside out, lowering inflammation and reversing chronic disease and dementia.

DON'T LET THE BAD BUGS BITE

We often think of sleep apnea as a disorder that afflicts adults, particularly those who are older and overweight.

It's true that people with low muscle tone and soft tissue around the airway are at a heightened risk for OSA. Common indicators include obesity, a BMI greater than 30, a large neck (sixteen inches for women, seventeen inches for men), enlarged tonsils, a large tongue, morning headaches, irritability, mood swings, depression, learning and memory difficulties, and sexual dysfunction. Risk of OSA rises with increase in body weight, active smoking, and age. Diabetics or borderline diabetics are up to three times more likely to have it.

Opportunities for prevention are available far earlier than we might think. By age three or four, kids can already be dealing with allergies that negatively affect their breathing, or other factors that make them "mouth breathers." They might snore, which we think is cute.

But it's not cute. For kids, even having one event an hour, one moment where their sleep is interrupted, can have a devastating impact. Interrupted sleep can affect the normal development of the prefrontal cortex, and then suddenly your child might receive a diagnosis of ADD or other disorders, which might have been prevented by ensuring uninterrupted, healthful sleep.

If, on the other hand, the prefrontal cortex develops the way it's supposed to, it yields positive neurobehavioral and neurocognitive results. This will affect the hippocampus, the brain center of emotion, memory, and the autonomic nervous system. A healthy prefrontal cortex can make your children far less susceptible to dementia and cognitive impairment later in life. It can even decrease the risk of anxiety and depression.

You wouldn't believe how many patients come to my practice with anxiety—and since many of them see me more often than their general practitioner, I'm the one they talk to about it. Dr. Gelb has gotten incredible results with his patients when it comes to anxiety.

"I can get rid of anxiety by 50 percent within two weeks," he says, "just by taking the airway that's being pinched and opening it up."

If you're anxious or depressed, you should always speak to a psychologist or psychiatrist. That said, I'm encouraged by the work doctors like Dr. Gelb are doing. Unblocking the airway could be another important tool in your tool kit when it comes to combatting mental illness, including drug-resistant anxiety and depression.

Good sleep habits and preventative measures can make a crucial difference in the well-being of your children, both now and in the future. Sleep is when the brain recharges. Human growth hormone is released at night, which is pivotal as your child grows and develops.

I believe you can prevent your kids from ever getting sleep apnea. And since men are more likely to suffer from sleep apnea than women, at a 3-to-1 ratio, just think of the positive impact this will have on your child's future relationships. Your sons will never become snorers like Tony, and your daughters will never become poor Beth, married to a man she has to exile to the guest room just to get a good night's sleep!

WHAT CAN YOU DO ABOUT IT?

The current and developing research on sleep apnea is very hopeful. Treatment of obstructive sleep apnea with continuous positive airway pressure (CPAP) and oral devices—more on those in a moment—improves levels of inflammatory markers. This is significant, considering atherosclerosis (the disease of the arteries we discussed in Chapter 4) is an inflammatory disease. OSA may be the link between atherosclerosis and periodontal disease that the dental community has been so interested in, since the association between these two conditions has been supported by evidence-based research.

Dr. Gelb has enjoyed phenomenal success in his practice. He and his team have developed a personalized treatment plan involving treatment of periodontal disease, laser periodontal therapy, and tray delivery system. This customized oral-hygiene plan also helps disrupt the colonization of bacteria and expose the hiding places of the bad bugs. Dr. Gelb's team of sleep experts monitor blood markers for inflammation, keeping track of how well they are doing to bring systemic inflammation down to ideal levels to keep patients at their healthiest.

At the heart of Dr. Gelb's work is the ACG™ AirwayCentric® System: the first fully integrated day-and-night oral-appliance approach to solving airway issues by integrating Airway and Sleep with TMJ. The system includes six appliances that complement the traditional ProSomnus [IA] Platform, including the Day and the Night.

The ACG™ Day is a lower milled repositioning device that covers the canines and establishes canine guidance while opening the airway during the day. It involves no clasps and is thinner lingually, allowing better speech—essential for a daytime appliance. It helps balance the nervous system and reduces pain while opening the airway, focusing on improving performance and energy levels while decreasing these symptoms.

The ACG™ Night appliance is an anti-retrusion appliance with either the same repositioning bite as the ACG™ Day or a slightly increased vertical and protrusive bite. The anterior guide ramp prevents the jaw from retruding. These appliances stop the lower jaw from dropping back at night, preventing a collapse of the airway during sleep. The main focus of the night appliances is to alleviate obstructive sleep apnea (OSA) and snoring and improve oxygenation, promoting more restorative sleep.

These are not your average oral appliances. While traditional nightguards may prevent wear of the teeth, they may or may not improve TMJ and clenching—and many actually worsen sleep-related breathing disorders (SRBD) and snoring. Dr. Gelb calls these ACG™ AirwayCentric® appliances "Nightguards 2.0." They won't close the airway and can alleviate clicking and locking, headaches, and neck pain. You may awaken more refreshed and with better focus and memory. And, of course, there are the huge long-term benefits of preventing cardiovascular disease and dementia.

At the end of the day, what if all we really need is a good night's sleep?

The following are some resources that might be helpful:

drmichaelgelb.com/nightguard-2-0/

drmichaelgelb.com/acg-system/

sleepfoundation.org

mayoclinic.com

chestnet.org

perioimplantadvisory.com

WHAT'S NEXT?

In the next chapter, we will discuss a condition in which a little extra weight is not only normal—it's exactly what you want. You'll also learn about how obesity and diabetes can be complicating factors for disease by aiding and abetting inflammation in the body.

If you want to know how periodontal disease can lead to pregnancy complications and preterm birth, read on.

CHAPTER 8

BABIES, BELLIES, AND BLOOD SUGAR

When Carolina and her husband, Sam, first became my patients, they wanted more than anything to have a baby. She was thirty-nine and he was forty-two, and they'd been trying to conceive for some time.

Carolina was one of those people who could make friends with anyone. She bonded quickly with my hygienist, who was also trying to get pregnant. They hit it off right away.

"We've been doing fertility treatments for the past two years," Carolina told her, "and I just don't think it's going to happen. I've always wanted to be a mother, and the thought of not being able to give Sam a son or daughter breaks my heart."

As my hygienist examined Caroline's mouth, she became clearly uncomfortable. The prognosis wasn't good. When she was asked, Carolina said her gums bled regularly when she flossed. She had high levels of bacteria in her mouth.

When we laid out a plan to get Carolina back on the path to oral health, she accepted the treatment plan without hesitation.

"Absolutely," she said. "If it means helping us improve our chances of getting pregnant, we'll do whatever it takes."

Six months later, Carolina told me about when she knew she was pregnant. She woke up and noticed her breasts were more tender than usual. For the next few days, she found herself urinating more frequently, and she felt bone tired in a way she'd never experienced before. Then she missed her period.

Carolina tried desperately not to get her hopes up. But she was trembling when she took the at-home pregnancy test. That evening, when Sam came home from work, she couldn't wait to tell him.

"It felt like a miracle," Carolina told me. "We knew God had answered our prayers."

I like telling this story, not only because it ends as a "happily ever after," but because it demonstrates the importance of understanding the oral-systemic health connection. We were able to heal the inflammation and infection in Carolina's mouth, helping pave the way for a healthy pregnancy. Nine months later, she and Sam welcomed Sam Jr.

There are other stories that don't end so happily. Women who do not maintain a healthy mouth during pregnancy can suffer severe and heartbreaking consequences. Though the science is still evolving, studies have suggested a link between inflammation and pregnancy complications such as preterm labor, preeclampsia (rise in blood pressure), and even stillbirth.

This is not something any pregnant couple should have to endure—which is why we need to talk about it, to ensure it never happens to you.

BACTERIA IS BAD FOR YOUR BABY

Here's a statistic that may surprise you: according to the World Health Organization, the United States ranks sixth among the top ten countries for premature births. Twelve percent—more than one in nine of all births—are preterm. That's half a million babies each year.

Dr. Yiping Han is a researcher at the College of Dental Medicine at Columbia University. Her focus is on oral microbiology; she studies how oral bacteria cause infections in the mouth and elsewhere in the body.

In 1996, a study was published providing the first evidence that women with periodontitis had a tendency to deliver premature and low-birth-weight babies. Since then, there have been a number of supporting epidemiological studies. In a paper published in the Journal of Dental Research, Dr. Han dug deep into the existing research. She concluded that "evidence is accumulating that oral bacteria may translocate directly into the pregnant uterus, causing localized inflammation and adverse pregnancy outcomes."

In layman's terms, this means that if bacteria from the mouth sneak into the blood circulation, they spray everywhere. Sound familiar? Some make their way into the uterus, where they can lead to infection, causing the sack of fluid to break prematurely, preterm labor, and—in worst-case scenarios—stillbirth.

To put it bluntly, it could kill the baby.

The findings from Dr. Han's studies are significant because they challenge the existing paradigm in the medical community. When doctors find an intrauterine infection, it's usually believed to originate in the vaginal tract. But Dr. Han's studies show that the bacteria may not come from the vaginal tract—and could very well come from the mouth through the bloodstream. In fact oral bacteria might account for anywhere between 10 to 30 percent of these infections.

Needless to say, the cost of bacteria invading a pregnant woman's uterus is incredibly high—physically, financially, and emotionally.

When a family loses a baby, it can be crushing. Grieving parents often wonder, Was this my fault? What did I do wrong? It breaks my heart to hear that question. I would love to prevent this kind of loss for as many parents as possible. It's a mission I strongly believe in—and one of the reasons I wanted to write this book.

Then there are couples like Carolina and Sam, who had a long, hard road to pregnancy in the first place. This infection can also infect the uterus in women not yet pregnant. It can make it exceedingly difficult to conceive in the first place, or kill the baby before it's even a known pregnancy; most miscarriages happen in the first twelve weeks.

Compounding the problem in some, there is strong science to support the thesis that women on fertility treatments may have trouble getting pregnant because the extra hormones given to stimulate fertility are absorbed into the estrogen receptors in their gums. If there is already bacterial infection present, the hormones can exacerbate it.

Intuitively, the oral-systemic connection makes sense. An infected uterus is a high-risk place for a tiny human to develop. A healthy mouth contributes to an environment that can allow for a healthy, successful pregnancy.

WHAT CAN YOU DO ABOUT IT?

We've all heard about strange pregnancy cravings, whether we've had them ourselves, known women who have had them, or seen them on TV. We joke about a mom-to-be needing her sardines and ice cream, but at the end of the day, she would do well to ditch the ice cream. The more frequently you give in to the craving for sugary snacks, the greater the chance of developing tooth decay. Studies have shown that the bacteria responsible for tooth decay pass from a mother to her child in utero. Not something you want your baby to inherit!

There are other aspects of pregnancy that make it more difficult to maintain good oral hygiene. For example, pregnant women with acid reflux are at a greater risk of tooth erosion and periodontal problems, as the acid begins to thin and wear away the enamel—the protective coating of the teeth—leaving them weakened. If you are experiencing acid reflux, you should talk to your dentist about ways of combatting these negative effects.

Increasingly, insurance companies are recognizing the value of healthy gums during pregnancy and are encouraging hygiene cleanings—and so do I.

Now let's talk about when you're carrying extra weight that's not a bun in the oven.

OBESITY, DIABETES, AND PERIODONTAL DISEASE: A VICIOUS CYCLE

We've touched briefly on obesity and diabetes as complicating factors of other diseases, but I wanted to add a few words here. Obesity is a medical condition in which excess body fat has accumulated to the extent that it may have an adverse effect on health. More than one third of US adults are obese. It is well known that obesity can increase the likelihood of sleep apnea, heart disease, Type 2 diabetes, and certain types of cancer.

In a study published in the Journal of Periodontology, obese individuals between the ages of eighteen and thirty-four were found to have a rate of periodontal disease that was 76 percent higher than individuals with a healthy weight. Obese patients have more tooth decay and more missing teeth. Since diet is partly to blame, I always encourage my obese patients to avoid sugary drinks, limit snacking, and eat a well-balanced diet. Bacteria love sugar as much as the rest of us, and when they feed on the sugars in food, they make acids. Over time, these acids destroy enamel, resulting in tooth decay.

Obesity and diabetes are often linked, insofar as obese men and women—especially those with belly fat—are at a higher risk for Type 2 diabetes. And to further connect the dots, gum disease is considered the sixth complication of diabetes. Patients with uncontrolled Type 2 diabetes are at a much higher risk for gum disease.

It's a vicious cycle because severe periodontal disease can increase blood sugar—and poor sugar control is what causes diabetes. Diabetes is a condition in which a person has high blood sugar (glucose). This occurs either because the insulin production is inadequate, or because the body's cells do not respond to insulin—or both.

Insulin's job is to pull glucose out of the blood and give it to tissues that need it. If you have an active periodontal infection, your blood-sugar level stays elevated, because when you have an infection of any kind in your body, it stimulates your liver to release sugar in an effort to fight off the infection.

Additionally, studies have shown that diabetics have a decreased ability to fight infections, including infection in the gums. This increases the bacterial load in the mouth, making gum inflammation worse. Together, these increase the likelihood that bacteria will enter the bloodstream to drive disease at distant sites.

We've all heard the nightmare stories of diabetic suffering, which can run the gamut from chronic fatigue to the loss of limbs. One diabetic patient of mine—a kind, compassionate attorney—always showed up for his appointments wrapped up in bandages. His body just couldn't heal itself. Every time he bumped or bruised himself, he'd have to ask his wife to dress the wound. And, of course, the same went for his teeth and gums. He knew he had periodontal disease, and he was prepared to do whatever it took to fight it. But his body just couldn't get healthy.

By now you probably see the circular nature of these conditions: diabetes can lead to periodontal disease, and periodontal disease can cause—and exacerbate—diabetes.

Researchers recently performed a study premised on the question "Which comes first, diabetes or periodontal disease?"

They followed the test subjects for years. One in particular stood out: a happy, healthy thirty-five-year-old woman with neither periodontal disease nor diabetes when the study began. About three and a half years later, she developed severe periodontal disease. So much bone was lost that her teeth actually migrated, and some of her back teeth were at risk of falling out.

What the researchers found was that, in the time between the two visits, this woman had also developed diabetes. If a patient has diabetes and also has periodontal disease, the periodontal disease makes diabetes worse—and vice versa.

This is a perfect example of the interaction between the mouth and the body. The oral-systemic link can work in both directions, a deleterious dance of cause and effect.

The following are some resources that might be helpful regarding pregnancy:

americanpregnancy.org
webmd.com/oral-health/dental-care-pregnancy
disabled-world.com
whattoexpect.com
dentalhealthandwellnessboston.com
perio.org/consumer

The following are some resources that might be helpful regarding obesity and diabetes:

webmd.com/oral-health
obesityaction.org
cdc.gov/obesity/data/adult.html
goodhealthstartshere.org
medicalnewstoday.com/info/diabetes
perio.org/consumer/mbc.diabetes.htm

WHAT'S NEXT?

We've talked about the relationship between inflammation and cardiovascular disease, dementia, cancers, sleep apnea, pregnancy complications, obesity, and diabetes.

We've talked about the vast and far-reaching consequences of periodontal disease on your health, happiness, and life.

But what are the broader implications of the oral-systemic link? As we move into a third era of health care, how do our choices affect our cities, our country, and our world?

CHAPTER 9

THE COST OF DOING NOTHING IS TOO GREAT

America is a wonderful country with so many opportunities and conveniences—so many that people even barely understand. But to be honest with you, I believe we have some work to do when it comes to keeping people healthy, happy, and free to live long, independent lives. Our current health-care system isn't about "health" at all—and that needs to change. We have a sick-care system.

Today's medical costs can be crushing. They certainly aren't competitive with other countries: health care in the United States is twice as expensive as in Europe, and four times as expensive as in Mexico, Japan, India, and China. Major companies have figured this out, which is why they've created incentive programs and wellness initiatives to encourage preventive care.

Our country has hit a pivotal inflection point. Health care has to become less expensive, and in my mind, the only way to accomplish that is to better maintain good health—and that starts with taking better care of our mouths.

In 2014, a landmark paper was published in the American Journal of Preventive Medicine. In the study—the first of its kind—researchers from the University of Pennsylvania conducted a comprehensive, five-year project in which they evaluated the claims of nearly 1.7 million patients covered by Highmark Health and United Concordia Dental. The researchers were looking specifically at patients with chronic medical conditions, and also pregnant women.

What they discovered was remarkable. Out of almost 1.7 million patients, 338,891 people who suffered from a chronic medical condition had also been diagnosed with periodontal disease. That's a solid 20 percent.

The researchers didn't stop there. They drilled down into the dollars and cents of the research, lasering in on patients who were actually treated for their gum disease. They found the annual financial savings to be impressive. People with coronary artery disease saved on average $1,090 yearly on their annual medical costs. Diabetics saved an average of $2,840 yearly. People who had suffered from a stroke saved a whopping $5,681. Women who were pregnant saved $2,433.

In my opinion, the savings in this study was significantly underestimated. The CDC (Centers for Disease Control and Prevention) estimates that 47.2 percent—nearly half of American adults—have periodontal disease. The fact that only 20 percent of the study participants had periodontal disease noted in their dental records proves the condition is severely underdiagnosed. If all those with periodontal disease had been identified and treated, the savings would have been much, much higher.

Thousands of dollars would be saved, simply by getting a healthier mouth.

HAVING A HEALTHY MOUTH IS SOMETHING TO BE PROUD OF

If the mouth is the gateway to complete health, then it follows that keeping our mouths healthy is the gateway to a stronger, healthier America.

But change doesn't happen on its own. There is a specially trained group of men and women in this country who will have to step forward and offer preventive care if we want to kick-start the revolution.

I'm one of them. Your friendly neighborhood dentist. Or, if you prefer something a little more fancy, "oral-systemic specialist."

I'm guessing that, before you read this book, dentists would not have been the first people to come to mind when you imagined solving our nation's health problems. But if you think about it, we dentists are in the ideal position to make a tremendous impact on our health-care system.

Generally, people are already in the habit of visiting the dentist every six months—way more often than the average American visits his or her primary-care physician. And as you now better understand, preventing disease is significantly less costly than trying to cure people once they have it. Considering the 162 diseases with early warning signs that can be detected in the mouth, we dentists may, in fact, be the perfect health professionals to prevent and reverse disease.

In other words, the system is already set up for the solution.

There has to be a contextual shift in how we think about the mouth. As Dr. Whitney says, we need to move into the third era of dentistry. Many dentists are still trapped in the old-school way of thinking. They subscribe to the "drill, fill, bill" mentality, or like so many physicians today, "treat it and beat it." We're trained to find the chief complaint and fix it. But that's a reactive care dentist. That's not the person who's going to be leading the revolution.

The times we're living in call for a new kind of dentistry—and to go with it, a new kind of dental team.

When we graduated from dentist school, we were taught to be problem solvers. In this new context of complete health, we understand that the body affects the mouth and the mouth affects the body.

For me personally, this shift in mind-set has allowed me to look at the whole patient. When I started asking people about their general medical history and their family history, I found that many of them hadn't been to see their physician for a checkup in years. That gave me the opportunity to engage in conversations with them about everything from smoking to exercise to getting that appointment with their primary-care physician to get a long-overdue physical.

When a patient comes into my practice, I don't just ask, "Is anything bothering you?" with the intent of fixing it and sending them on their merry way. I look at their health from a wider scope. When I'm treating their periodontal disease, I'm also looking for signs and symptoms of other diseases or conditions. I encourage them to go see their general practitioner to discuss the concerns we raised in the dental office.

I treat the whole person, not just the mouth. My patients see my team and me as more than just a dental office. We care about their total body health and well-being.

Am I trying to replace physicians? Not at all. I want to partner with my fellow medical professionals. If the mouth is the first line of defense, that means I have a lot of responsibility to keep you healthy. I have valuable information about your health that I can share with your primary-care physician or other doctors—and I don't take that responsibility lightly. Neither do my hygienists, who are critical to providing the best care we can offer.

We are assuming our needed role in the integrated model of health care. When I think of the future of our country as Complete Health Dentistry® takes root, I have a very clear vision. I imagine the full spectrum of health-care practitioners coming together to provide you with the very best in holistic, integrated care. I imagine physicians understanding and embracing the importance of the oral cavity as a powerful gateway to complete health, not a separate island cut off from the rest of our body.

I imagine a world in which the public government, insurance carriers, physicians, dentists, hygienists, pharmacists, dieticians, and all other health professionals understand dentistry as the first line of defense against sickness and debilitating disease.

I imagine patients who are excited to assume ownership of their own health, taking proactive and preventive measures to ensure they live a long, healthy life.

That's the reason our office practices Complete Health Dentistry®. I believe dentists can change the world.

But I can't do it alone. In order to turn the tide as we move boldly into the third era of health care, there's one more person who plays a pivotal role.

You.

CHAPTER 10

THE COMPLETE HEALTH DENTISTRY® TRANSFORMATION

Professional dentistry's been around for almost a century and a half. And for all that time, dentists have been pushing away the tongue in order to see the mouth. They've literally been overlooking the body, forgetting that gums and teeth are attached to people.

But that's finally changing. Complete Health® dentists are taking a holistic view of oral health care—a view that captures whole bodies and whole lives. We're looking at everything from the tip of your tongue to the back of your throat, and we're using our discoveries to improve the way you eat, the way you sleep, and the way you live.

I didn't start my dental practice so that I could fix fillings and whiten teeth. I started it to help people. And it doesn't matter whether those people been prioritizing health care their whole lives or they're just beginning—whether they're fit as fiddles or battling chronic conditions like diabetes, hypertension, and heart disease. At my practice, we're committed to serving everyone.

And we've put our money where our mouths are, investing in transformative new dental technology. Our digital x-rays cut radiation exposure down by 80 percent; our CEREC machines slash crown-creation time down from weeks to minutes; and our cone beam x-rays have literally saved lives.

But, as my newborn son's doctor told me years ago, health care isn't about healing people. It's about helping people heal themselves. So if you want to achieve and sustain good health, you need to take the lead by doing three things:

#1: GET YOUR FRIDGE IN ORDER

Many of us have bought into the idea that our families have genetic predispositions toward a wide range of chronic illnesses. But much of the time, we mistake nurture for nature, blaming the genes that we've inherited instead of the habits that we've inherited. And some of the most important habits we pass on are those that relate to diet. Remember this: the diet on which you raise your children will be the diet on which they raise their children.

Lately, we've been hearing a lot about the rise of ADHD among children. We hear that kids can't sit still any more, and that they can't focus. Prescriptions for Ritalin-type medications have become more and more common.

But if you walked my route to work in the morning, you would see corner store after corner store full of children spending their breakfast money on sodas and candy bars. You wouldn't blame learning challenges and behavioral problems on ADHD. You'd blame them on sugar.

Sugar has become the most accessible, most abused drug in America. In addition to wreaking havoc on our moods and our focus, it lowers our immunity to illness, stimulates oral bacterial growth, and promotes inflammation, tooth decay, and gum disease.

And it's everywhere. Our processed foods are chalk full of all sorts of sugars, from honey to cane sugar to high fructose corn syrup. But a sugar by any other name is just as bad for you.

Still, I'm not suggesting that you eliminate sugar altogether. I'm encouraging you to take a closer look at your diet and search for places where you can make reductions.

To do that, you'll want to start by collecting some data with a food diary. For one week, every time you put food into your mouth, write down what you had. And be as detailed as possible. Don't just write "coffee with sugar"; note how much sugar you're taking. How many pats of butter go on your bread? And what kind of bread is it? These details will become crucial when you start experimenting with changes to your diet, which is what you'll want to do next.

Once you've finished a week of journaling, start experimenting with changes. And do it gradually. If you throw out all of your food and vow to eat nothing but kale and carrots for the rest of your life, you're bound to relapse. Instead, try to find little ways that you can begin transforming your diet, gradually weaning yourself off of sugary, fatty, and processed foods.

If you're eating a bowl of ice cream every night, try moving over to twice a week. If you're putting three packets of sugar in your coffee, try moving over to two for a week. Then one.

And start looking at ingredients when you shop. Low-sugar tomato sauce looks and tastes just like its high-sugar counterparts. But unlike those counterparts, low-sugar tomato sauce won't slowly kill you and your family.

Likewise, beware of foods that sound healthier than they are. Cartons of orange juice promise that lots of vitamin C will help your child's immune system, but serving a child fruit juice is basically like hooking them up to a sugar IV. The same goes for sports drinks, which we've come to associate with athleticism despite the fact that they're full of tooth-dissolving sugars and kidney-killing food dyes.

So instead of putting that orange juice or apple juice in your cart, try heading over to the produce section and loading up on the actual fruits that those juices masquerade as. Instead of giving your little athletes sports drinks, encourage them to hydrate with water. They can get their electrolytes from fruit, seeds, and nuts.

When you're first starting out, studying ingredients and modifying your shopping list might add some time to your grocery routine, but you'll quickly get to know which items are which. You'll be back to speed-shopping in no time. And you'll probably be able to shop faster than you ever could before. Because you won't have sugar slowing you down.

#2: GET YOUR BED IN ORDER

Absolutely nothing you do to get healthy is going to matter if you aren't sleeping well. And I'm talking about both quantity and quality. At minimum, we all need to get six hours of sleep. And that has to be good, undisturbed sleep.

To that end, cut out food and alcohol before bed, otherwise they're going to pester you all night. Make sure you're sleeping in a temperate room—one that's neither too hot nor too cold. And when bedtime comes, shut off all your devices. You don't want anything waking you up, and you don't want that electronic glow lighting the room. Silence and darkness are your friends.

Now, unfortunately, even under ideal conditions, many of my patients have trouble getting a full night's sleep because they suffer from sleep apnea. So if you aren't sleeping well, and if you're experiencing excessive daytime fatigue, forgetfulness, or acid reflux, consider the possibility that you might be struggling with a sleep disorder. If you have hypertension or diabetes, you need to get a sleep test as well. (If you have a partner, check in with them to find out whether you're snoring. That could mean it's an airway blockage keeping you up at night.) There is even an app you can get on your phone to find out if you might possibly snore at night.

Now, if you do have sleep apnea, don't worry too much. Just bring it up with your dentist. Of all your health care providers, we spend the most time in your mouth, so we're the ideal people to talk to about airway ailments. We can often determine whether you have sleep apnea just by studying the shape of your mouth and the size of your tongue.

For those who do have mild or moderate sleep apnea, we work closely with your general physician, and we can, in our office, fabricate a simple dental appliance to help open your airway at night. If you have severe apnea, we'll refer you to a sleep physician and they will usually prescribe either a CPAP machine, which will help you breathe while you sleep, or a simple dental appliance to open up your airway.

#3: GET YOUR TEETH IN ORDER

Finally, brush effectively, floss effectively, and visit your dentist. Ideally, you should be brushing after every meal—especially before bed. That ensures that sugar and other bacteria-breeding foods don't get trapped in your teeth. And if you can't brush after a daytime meal, I'd recommend that you rinse out your mouth with water.

But simply brushing and flossing aren't enough. You need to do those things effectively so that you're actually removing plaque and bacteria. If you don't get the angles right, you could end up leaving big gaps in your oral hygiene.

Unfortunately, there aren't one-size-fits-all directions for effective brushing. Every person's mouth and dental history is different. Different shapes require different strategies and so do different dental appliances like crowns and bridges. That's one of the reasons why it's crucial that you visit a dentist at least twice a year. They'll take a look around and work with you to find the best daily care strategies for your mouth.

But, as you'll know by now, there's more to dentist visits than oral hygiene. There are more than a hundred different diseases that can we can detect just by taking a look inside your mouth—diseases that need to be caught early if we're going to beat them.

Most people see a general doctor once a year. Maximum. As a result, dentists have really become this country's primary care physicians, checking in with patients twice yearly to evaluate their health and keep a wary eye for red flags.

If you don't have a dentist yet, please find one. And be sure it's a good one—one who will help you celebrate the decision to get healthy, not one who will put you down because you didn't do it sooner. Make sure it's the kind of dentist who's going to look at you as a whole person, not just a set of thirty-two teeth.

If you have any questions about the process, feel free to reach out to me and my office. We'll be happy to help you navigate your oral health journey. And if you're in the New York area, we'd be delighted to set up an appointment. You can find us online at www.morningsidedentalcare.com or reach us by email at info@morningsidedentalcare.com.

Complete Health Dentistry® isn't just for elites. In fact, quite the contrary: it's only the super-rich who can afford traditional health care. Because the first rule of medical economics is that treatment costs infinitely more than prevention. If you can catch problems early, you won't have to invest in costly surgical procedures or extortionate prescription medicines.

But even if the money doesn't matter to you, I hope that your life does—your work, your friends, your family. You owe it to them to get healthy, to stay healthy, and to help them get healthy too.

All that health begins with the mouth. It begins with the smile.

Our smiles tell the world the best things about us. Which is why it breaks my heart to see so many broken smiles—smiles that hold people back from landing dream jobs and finding their perfect mates. For everyone I've ever cared for—from family members like my son to patients like Jeffrey Jackson—it's their smiles I remember most. And, to this day, it's their smiles that protect them.

At the beginning of this book, I brought up the poetry of Tupac Shakur. I suspect that he probably wasn't thinking about the oral-systemic health connection when he wrote his verses. He may not have known that oral health care has the capacity to prevent strokes, diabetes, cancers, kidney disease, Alzheimer's, and heart disease. But that doesn't change the literal and figurative truth of the words he wrote—the words I live by and the words I hope you'll live by too:

The power of a smile can heal a frozen heart.

NOTES

Breslow, Dr. Lester, "*Health Measurement in the Third Era of Health.*" Am J Public Health. 2006 January; 96(1): 17–19.

Pussinen PJ, Jousilahti P, Alfthan G, Palosuo T, Asikainen S, Salomaa V. "*Antibodies to periodontal pathogens are associated with coronary heart disease*". Arterioscler Thromb Vasc Biol. 2003; 23: 1250–1254

Pussinen PJ, Alfthan G, Rissanen H, Reunanen A, Asikainen S, Knekt P. "*Antibodies to periodontal pathogens and stroke risk.*" Stroke. 2004; 35: 2020–2023

Kozarov EV, Dorn BR, Shelburne CE, Dunn WA, Progulske-Fox A. "*Human Atherosclerotic Plaque Contains Viable Invasive Actinobacillus actinomycetemcomitans and Porphyromonas gingivalis.*"Arteriosclerosis, Thrombosis, and Vascular Biology. 2005;25:e17-e18.

Bale, Dr. Brad and Doneen, Dr. Amy, "*The Vital Importance of the Mouth-Body Connection.*" http://oralsystemiclink.net/patients/profile/the-vital-importance-of-the-mouth-body-connection: April 20, 2017.

https://www.alz.org/alzheimers-dementia/facts-figures

http://www.alzinfo.org/understand-alzheimers/dementia/

https://newsblogdrexeledu/2016/02/10do-infections-causeazheimers-disease/

Miklossy, Judith. Neuroinflammation. 2011 Aug 4;8:90. doi: 10.1186/1742-2094-8-90. https://www.ncbi.nlm.nih.gov/pubmed/21816039

Allen et al., *"Alzheimer's Disease: A Novel Hypothesis Integrating Spirochetes, Biofilm, and the Immune System."* J Neuroinfectious Diseases 2016, 7:1. http://dx.doi.org/10.4172/2314-7326.1000200.

Wheeler, Mark. *"Memory loss associated with Alzheimer's reversed for first time."* October 2, 2014. http://newsroom.ucla.edu/releases/memory-loss-associated-with-alzheimers-reversed-for-first-time

Ha, N.H., Woo, B.H., Kim, D.J. et al. Tumor Biol. (2015) 36: 9947. https://doi.org/10.1007/s13277-015-3764-9

http://www.who.int/pmnch/media/news/2012/preterm_birth_report/en/index3.html

Han, Yiping. *"Oral health and adverse pregnancy outcomes—what's next?"* J Dent Res. 2011 Mar;90(3):289-93. doi: 10.1177/0022034510381905. Epub 2010 Nov 1.

https://www.webmd.com/baby/understanding-miscarriage-basics#1

Al–Zahrani MS, Bissada NF, Borawskit EA. *Obesity and periodontal disease in young, middle aged and older adults.* J Periodontol. 2003;74:610–5

https://www.unitedconcordia.com/docs/united%20concordia%20oral%20health%20whitepaper.pdf

P.I. Eke, B.A. Dye, L. Wei, G.O. Thornto-Evans, R.J. Genco. *"Prevalence of Periodontitis in Adults in the United States: 2009 and 2010."* Volume: 91 issue: 10, page(s): 914-920. Article first published online: August 30, 2012; Issue published: October 1, 2012. http://journals.sagepub.com/doi/abs/10.1177/0022034512457373.